Dr. Stephen K Fairley

Cover & book illustration by
Harry McGlone

Edited by:
Dianne Stallan

Printing:
Prime Print Pty Ltd

Chapters

INTRODUCTION

When most of you think about getting old and the remedies to delay your inevitable death, you picture someone going through life and getting stuck in old age for a long time, just before they die, "I don't want to live the life of, or look like a person who is 110 years old." You say appropriately "I don't want that, it's not for me, I'm happy to die when my time is up."

This concept could not be further from the truth or the point of the book. The book is not about staying old, it is about staying young. We are not interested in prolonging the life of people who are old with a relatively poor quality of life. The aim of this book is to keep people young and even more importantly than that it is to keep them disease free so they have the maximum potential to live happy productive and fulfilling lives. That is why we use the term health span not lifespan.

It looks almost certain that there are drugs coming

which will dramatically prolong people's lives but they are not here yet. The discussion in this book centres on important discoveries which appear to control the rate at which we age and at which we get age related diseases. Age and most common diseases are very closely intertwined and sometimes there is a "chicken and egg" issue where it is not possible to say which causes the other. They blend into the same thing. The hope here is that we can prevent or delay age related decline and specific age related diseases such as heart disease, type 2 diabetes, dementia, cancer and many others.

To achieve this, you need to be an active player in the game and have some understanding of the processes involved. Diet is one of the most important issues and yes again, I feel you have been told all the wrong things by the medical profession and other well-meaning health professionals over the last 60-70 years. They may all have the best intentions but I think their advice lacks the evidence necessary to back it up. It is never too late to make changes however. There are also medications freely available today, which may be beneficial here with minimal significant side effects. I will discuss the evidence for considering these medications and you can then discuss with your doctor if you feel this approach is appropriate for you. I would not necessarily start with medication.

The dietary changes should be the first line and these

are simple and easy to make. You just need to know what to do.

CHAPTER 1

Why Do We Need To Age?

The only reason life still exists on this planet is because it can rejuvenate itself. This process allows it to keep pace with an ever-changing environment. Living things do this by making new copies of themselves. Every time this occurs there is the potential for errors or mutations occurring in the genetic material controlling the features of the next generation. These errors occur by chance – like rolling dice - and most of them make the offspring less likely to survive. As a consequence, most of these new "mutants" die off.

Every now and then however you get a lucky number on the dice and the new mutant of a species picks up something which makes it more rather than less likely to survive. If you are a small fish which is at risk of being eaten by larger fish, and an accidental change or mutation occurred with replication of the DNA controlling your colour, this would make you either more or less likely to survive. If this change made you more closely resemble the colour of the background seaweed in which you hide from the larger fish you would consequently be less likely to be eaten and more likely to survive. If your colour changed so that you stood out, you would not last long. If you are more likely to survive you are also more likely to get to breed and to pass on this colour change to the next generation of fish, who are also blessed with better camouflage, as are their offspring. This process plays over and over millions of times until this fish species and the seaweed are the same colour. Each change only needs to be tiny but these tiny changes add up because this game of chance is played out so many times.

This process has shaped the evolution of all forms of life from tiny bacteria and yeasts to complex large forms of life such as dinosaurs or mammals roaming the planet today. These mammals include the species Homo sapiens or if you like humans like you and me.

So why does this mean we must die? Couldn't we all just go on living forever? Well this issue is also part of the equation which determines the likelihood of a species surviving. The issue here is availability of resources to keep the species alive and breeding. The more individuals there are the less food there is to go around and in times of famine the whole species would die off. The only individuals of the species which really matter - to the process of evolution and long term survival of the species - are those that can breed and produce offspring, ensuring survival of the species. Once an individual within a species gets past the age of reproduction (and caring for offspring until these offspring can fend for themselves) they are a burden on the survival of the species as, not an asset. The longer they live past this age of reproduction and nurturing of offspring, the more likely the species is to die out. The old members of the species are in competition with the younger breeders for food and other resources. Again, when this is played out millions of times the life expectancy of individuals within a species becomes the optimal for overall survival of this species. It does not matter if this species is of flies or elephants. All the species who got this wrong in the past are now fossils in rocks. They have all died out. This is how evolution works. None of their descendants inhabit the planet today.

If we accept Homo sapiens have only been in existence on this planet for about 150,000 years we have not had much time to play this out. During most of this time we were hunter gatherers living in caves or in the open. Our life span was only about 30-40 years. This meant breeding as soon as it was possible, presumably as teenagers. One assumes there was also a survival advantage to the group in our living a bit beyond the breeding years as our young take so long to become independent. Hunter gathering is hard and dangerous work, presumably one had to be able to run fast and climb trees and the younger members of the group would have been the best suited to this. They were also the ones doing the breeding. This meant the older members would presumably have had to stay home and look after the vulnerable offspring. Once the offspring were independent the sooner the older members of the group died the better for the survival of the group - the fewer the mouths to feed. There is nothing fair, forgiving or caring about evolution it is just about maths and likelihood of species survival. The maths of probability. This determined our life expectancy. Living in the wild is much more dangerous than living today and once your physical capability and senses started to fail you didn't last long. Just enough time to get your grandchildren independent. These grandchildren would have grown up much faster than they do today - they had to.

This pressure for survival of the species, or if you like evolution, has built into us a clock (or clocks) which determine how rapidly we age and consequently our life expectancy. We must outsmart this clock and the processes running it if we are to optimise life expectancy, stay young and avoid age related disease. We must understand what makes this clock(s) tick if we are to be able to make these adjustments to it.

CHAPTER 2

The Theories Of Ageing

Mankind has been worrying about why we age and what we can do about this for thousands of years. In the process, we have come up with more than 300 different theories of ageing, most of them in the last few decades. Now before you panic and throw this book in the rubbish – I have no intention of discussing them all. Such a discussion would bore us both to death literally. I do think you need a general overview of these theories however to be able to have logical discussions with others and to interpret the scientific literature if you do further reading.

The trouble with these theories is that they all seem to have holes in them. Ageing is likely a very complex process and it may well be that no single theory or hypothesis can cover all the bases. In other words, don't necessarily regard the different theories as mutually exclusive, there may be part truths in many of them which need to be put together to arrive at a unifying hypothesis which best explains the process of ageing. We are not there yet by any means. My problem with all these theories is that they do not predict the future, in experimental terms.

Let me give you an example to explain this concept. Sir Isaac Newton is said to have been watching an apple fall off a tree when he came up with the theory of gravity. Newton's law of gravitation states that every particle in the universe attracts every other particle with a force which is directly proportional to the product of their masses and inversely proportional to the square of the distance between them. This is less complicated than it sounds if you stop and think about it. It explains the apparent weight of things in your environment or if you like the gravitational force exerted by the earth upon them. It explains why a handful of lead is much heavier than a handful of feathers. It explains why in a perfect vacuum the handful of feathers and the handful of lead fall at the same rate and would hit the ground at the same time no matter what the height you dropped them from. You can test this theory over and over and over again – it always works! It predicts the future result of your experiment. Every time you do the experiment properly the law of gravity is 100% accurate in predicting the outcome of that experiment. In scientific terms this makes it a law of science, rather than just a theory.

Now go and test the theories of ageing, perhaps by adding more oxygen to a container you are growing worms in and see if they die at a younger age and if so how much younger – as some theories of ageing would predict. You know what? It never works properly! In other words when you test these ageing theories they never work like a true scientific theory, they all have holes in them. None of them properly or truly explain the theory of ageing. They remind me of psychiatrists and psychologists trying to predict human behaviour with their theories and models. They get it wrong most of the time because they do not understand how the mind works. It is far too complicated. If they did fully understand how the mind works they could accurately predict human behaviour. They may be right occasionally but their accuracy is nothing like Newton's. The theories of ageing would be better termed the hypotheses of ageing.

None the less you do need to have a basic understanding of the biological theories of ageing as they all probably contain some truths. Generally speaking, the theories fall into two main categories. That ageing is programmed into our genes and controlled by them, or that ageing is the result of wear and tear.

The **Programmed theories** suggest ageing is embedded in our genetic makeup. Ageing could simply be a process resulting from turning on and off certain genes, a bit like your passing through puberty for example. Genes are switched on and off to start and finish puberty and the same is possibly true to bring on ageing and age related diseases.

There are those who think this biological clock works through hormones and these theories are called endocrine theories. There is no doubt that the signalling of certain hormones or chemical messengers is involved in ageing, particularly insulin and insulin like growth factors, both of which I will discuss in more detail later in the book. They are right, these chemical messengers are very important in the ageing process.

There are also those who believe the programmed theory operates through the immune system, the so called immunological theories. They would have you believe that many bodily functions such as avoiding cancer and nasty infections is dependent on a good immune surveillance system and when this starts to fail – as it does progressively as you age – then you get into trouble. They are also right on all counts above, the immune system is best in adolescence and progressively declines throughout life. The immune system also seems to become dysregulated as you age, it seems to lose track of who or what exactly it should be shooting at. This results in it being inappropriately switched on causing continuous low grade inflammation – rather than simply being switched on when it is needed to fight a specific infection such as the measles virus. This continuous low grade inflammation is strongly associated with western diseases such as diabetes, cardiovascular disease, cancer and Alzheimer's disease coming on at an earlier age. I think this process of inappropriate switching on of the immune system is more likely related to environmental factors than being programmed in your genes but perhaps there is an element of truth in both options, it does become more of an issue with ageing.

The **wear and tear, damage or error theories** are perhaps easier for many of you to accept because it is what happens in the environment all around you. As your car ages with wear so do the tyres, the engine and all the moving parts. Eventually it ends up as landfill (as you will too) and you need to go out and get another one. A pity we can't do that with you.

Again, you can break down these wear and tear theories into different groups where scientists try to explain why you do "wear out and fall to bits", as my father would say. One relates to the rate of living theory. This is based on the fact that the greater an organism's metabolic rate or oxygen consumption, the shorter is its life and generally in nature this is correct. These organisms tend to get everything done more quickly and so don't really have the need to hang around, at least in evolutionary terms. If you try to apply this theory to people you would predict that a thin person who exercises a lot with a consequent high metabolic rate and more rapid oxygen consumption would die sooner than a sloth who never gets off the couch and prefers to watch other people play sport rather than participate personally. We all know the reverse of what this theory predicts is actually the truth. This theory falls well short of Newton and his apples when you test it in real life.

The crosslinking theory focuses on the protein component of your body, these proteins are the blocks you are built from and they also perform many bodily processes. Protein is rapidly turned over and reproduced and it is in chains of subunits called amino acids. If these chains get tangled or stick together they can "clog up" your working environment in the cell. It is a bit like trying to work in a workshop where there is litter everywhere rather than one that is neat and tidy. Trying to vacuum the carpet in an adolescent's bedroom would be another good example – there are things all over the floor and you are better just to throw your arms in the air, give up and close the bedroom door. Better still give the vacuum cleaner to the adolescent, but you know in reality it will never get used. More and more things will accumulate on the floor of that bedroom. This accumulated rubbish in the cell occurs with increasing age and age related diseases. For example, in Alzheimer's disease we call the rubbish neurofibrillary tangles or amyloid plaques which litter the brain cells and are possibly important in bringing about their dysfunction and demise with subsequent dementia in the sufferer.

The free radical theory has been around since the 1950s and is based on the body's need to use oxygen.

By necessity free radicals or single oxygen molecules with a free electron are an unavoidable result of the use of oxygen in any chemical reaction and these free radicals are like loose cannons, they damage things around them. They react with the nearest thing they can find and this can be protein, RNA or DNA (our genes). This damage is cumulative with time and will eventually if unchecked, lead a cell to stop functioning. It clearly cannot be the whole story however as is evident in the example given above in the rate of metabolism theory - exercise does not correlate inversely with lifespan. By necessity we also have many defences and repair mechanisms against free radicals.

The DNA damage theory suggests that every time a cell replicates, as most of our cells need to do to keep us alive, there is the potential for errors, where the wrong chain link or so called nucleotide is placed in the chain being copied from the original. The cell has mechanisms to correct this error but some get missed, and these missed errors are passed on to future cells in subsequent divisions leading to DNA with multiple errors in it and subsequent loss of function and cell death. Clearly if it was this simple life would not exist on the planet at all – it would all have died off because of errors made in replicating. This means the germ cells, the sperm in males and eggs in women must be protected from this process so they can pass on good quality DNA to future generations and ensure survival of the species.

You have to start somewhere in science or scientific processes. There probably are some elements of truth in any of the theories above and the truth may be a complicated mix of many of them. The problems as I see them are firstly; any single one of these theories fails dismally when it comes to predicting the outcome of experiments done in the laboratory when you try to prove their validity. These experiments are done on unfortunate "lesser" forms of life than ourselves. Secondly; they do not really offer any useful therapeutic implications we can use. It is alright to say oxygen is harmful and may cause ageing with or without discussion involving free radicals, but what is the alternative! You can try holding your breath and give up oxygen but then this discussion becomes somewhat academic.

I stress again I am a practical person not a theorist. I am looking for things that make a difference even if we don't fully understand the mechanisms involved. When you go looking there are many interesting things out there with therapeutic implications we can use. This book will focus on the areas where there is scientific evidence to back up claims and where you can do things that are likely to make a difference in the health span of your life.

We have been aware since the 1930s that fasting or calorie restricting laboratory animals prolongs their lifespan. The proponents of many of the theories above will claim their theory explains why this is so but I beg to differ and will offer an alternative view albeit one which probably overlaps. I will discuss this in more detail in the section on diet and m-TOR.

Another fascinating observation in ageing relates to **Telomeres**. If this sounds like Greek to you that is because it is. The word is derived from the Greek "telos" meaning end and "meros" meaning part. It refers to the end part of a chromosome. Remember our chromosomes are made up of long chains of DNA molecules called nucleotides. These chains dictate the template for life itself and almost all the functions of our cells. These molecules are critical for life and they need to be protected. One of their protective components is the caps on the ends of the chains. These repeating sequences of the nucleotides TTAGGG do not convey any useful information, unlike the genes in the chromosome proper. Every time a cell reproduces it must make a new copy of the chromosomes, for the new cell. The enzyme complex which replicates the DNA chain never quite gets to the end of the chain and consequently a bit drops off, in other words the next chain is shorter. This does not usually matter as the bit left off is from the telomere on the end – and is not one of your genes.

After somewhere around 40-80 cellular divisions, in most tissues, you run out of telomeres and at that point the division stops. The cell is unable to further divide because it would be chopping off bits of the active DNA which would result in its death. It is said to be in a senescent state.

This means one would expect your telomeres to progressively shorten with age as your cells divide and this is indeed what occurs. The length of your telomeres would also predict your life expectancy and to some extent they do. When you ran out of telomeres you would die and generally this seems to be the case.

The implications are that each cell has a biological division clock setting up a maximal number of allowable divisions. The obvious conclusion is that if there was a way of preventing the shortening of these telomeres we may be able to live forever, with immortal cells which could go on dividing forever. There is always the argument of association and causation not being the same thing. This may be a fly in the ointment of your wonderful new theory. In other words, the shortening of telomeres which unquestionably occurs with ageing is not the cause of ageing, it is simply a marker for ageing.

The jury is still out on this case and we are not sure what to believe. There remains the possibility that drugs may protect or re vitalise telomeres and delay or stop ageing, but they have not been marketed yet. There is a herbal extract from the Chinese herb Astragalus root, named TA-65, which can indeed lengthen telomeres however it is expensive to produce as it needs to be concentrated and when tested in female mice did not lead to any prolongation of life span, despite lengthening telomeres.

There is an enzyme in your cells that can lengthen the telomeres and it is called telomerase. The TA-65 acts by activating this enzyme. Telomerase is permanently active in some cells, which must indeed be able to live or propagate forever, our germ cells - the sperm and eggs from which we are made. Otherwise we would all die off in a few generations. These germ cells express the enzyme telomerase but almost all other cells in our body lose the enzyme expression after we are born. These somatic cells still have the genetic code there to make telomerase, as we have the same DNA in all cells, it is just in the off position and not active.

There is a good theoretical reason for switching off telomerase in most cell lines and it relates to that scary word cancer. You have an inbuilt anti-cancer mechanism. If any cell in your body loses control and goes haywire with respect to growth and division, as cancers do, it gets stopped dead in its tracks when it gets to that magical 40 odd cellular divisions and dies off. The only time it will be able to go beyond this is if it switches on the gene to make the telomerase and repair its telomeres. You guessed it, this is exactly what cancer cells do to enable them to become immortal and keep dividing until they kill their host.

This leads us to the assumption that if you could

inhibit telomerase you would do very little harm, as most cells do not express it, and you may inhibit cancer growth. There is a lot of research going on here but there is one problem. I have oversimplified this a bit. Some cell lines need to be able to divide more than the limit of 40-80 times. They probably include the skin which is continuously shedding, the lining of the gut and the bone marrow, which makes your blood cells and immune cells. These cells need telomerase to keep dividing and to keep you alive, if you blocked it here you would be in trouble. Scientists need to be able to selectively block the enzyme in cancer cells and they are working on this as fast as they can.

So, the whole concept of telomerase and telomeres is a fascinating one and there may be effective therapies for ageing and cancer coming out of research here but just like you have to say to the kids in the back seat of the car, "we are not there yet!".

Keep watching this space.

CHAPTER 3

Ageing and disease, are they the same thing?

The short answer is yes, at least for the diseases which matter most in Western societies.

There are clearly a number of different types or classes of disease or if you like things which make you unwell and put you at risk of dying. If we are discussing the important diseases in the last 149.5 thousand of the 150 thousand years we have walked on this planet, then a large proportion of humans would have died from infectious disease and from trauma. The world was a much more dangerous place. Many of us died long before we were programmed to by the other evolutionary forces discussed in chapter 1.

Times have changed however. We rarely die from the things we once did. The process of evolution as we knew it in the past has largely stopped. Our environment no longer directly controls the likelihood of our survival, and consequently our breeding, with the passage of our genes to future generations. We have been interfering with this process with things like modern medicine and modern engineering which now protect us from the threats of the past. From the threats which shaped our evolution and the length of our lives amongst other things.

To some extent this leaves us floundering in a "brave new world" for want of a better term, and nothing to do with the book of the same name. A whole host of new diseases have come in to fill the void left by our eradicating the old diseases. The new diseases are largely metabolic and degenerative in nature. As mentioned already, my father who was also a medical practitioner would say "you're just getting older and falling to bits!" in describing this to patients, a term some of you will know I tend to use as well. It is not entirely correct however. To some extent the "falling to bits" determines the "getting older" but it's not all related to simple wear and tear with subsequent failure of componentry. In many diseases, we may have the chicken and egg the wrong way around. Sorry this concept is a bit complex and confusing and I am not for a second suggesting we fully understand it.

Let me use a car engine as an example again to demonstrate this point. Every time you drive your car around the engine wears out a bit. You know as well as I do it will not last forever. If everything is optimised, in other words it does not get too hot, it is well lubricated... then hopefully it will last a long time, perhaps even for as long as the manufacturer told you it would! This is its potential lifespan.

Then you have the car serviced and at the service they put the wrong oil in the engine, so it is not properly lubricated, gets too hot and wears out more rapidly. It wears out and starts to die long before it should have done, long before it gets to its potential lifespan. In your case, the wrong oil in the engine is what we call a "modern lifestyle" which includes our diet, exercise and other things as diverse as the types and number of bacteria in your gut. All these things have an effect on your potential lifespan. They express themselves as the common diseases in western society such as things like the metabolic syndrome and possibly autoimmune diseases. Autoimmune diseases including allergies we do not really understand possibly relates to our environment having been "too clean' while we were growing up. Autoimmune disease does rob some of us of our potential lifespan but is numerically much less important than the metabolic syndrome.

The metabolic syndrome is well described in prior publications and is a disease we can do something about. We do understand some of the contributing factors. Under the umbrella of the metabolic syndrome I include numerous common illnesses such as cardiovascular disease, most of the common cancers, type 2 diabetes and dementia to name a few. These are the usual cause of death of most people in our modern societies and there is the potential to both prevent the disease and delay the death. There is no such thing as dying from natural causes, as a doctor you cannot put "natural causes" on a death certificate, it would be rejected and sent back to be filled out properly. Everyone dies from something.

The issue here is that these now common diseases, which will result in the deaths of most of us, and the process of ageing, are intricately interrelated. The diseases are much more likely to occur with increasing age, no argument. Just like an engine will wear out eventually. The problem is when you put the wrong oil in your engine these diseases occur much earlier than they need to, robbing you of potential life span and contributing to your premature death.

I know, I know, you don't want to live forever! I have heard this many times, since the poor choice of the title for a previous publication "Do you want to live to be 100?". Stop and think for me now. This argument is as much about quality of life as it is about quantity of life and I am offering you both. The health span as opposed to life span, is what we are primarily aiming to improve on. This is the period of your life during which you are fully functioning and free of disease. Able to enjoy your life to the fullest and hopefully contribute maximally to the care and wellbeing of others such as your dependents, or those not as well off as you are.

You have the choice of being admitted to a nursing home at the age of 70 with dementia and wearing nappies for the second time in your life. You soil these regularly and some other family member or nurse must change them for you. Otherwise you unintentionally use the floor or a chair as the toilet. You take 23 tablets per day, none of which you can name and which your nurse dutifully dishes out to you and watches you swallow. You don't remember any of your family or friends, you just sit there dribbling, wearing a bib and staring blankly into space. You have forgotten how to talk. You cannot walk because your left leg has been removed because of the arterial disease associated with your long history of diabetes. You have now suffered what I would call TOTAL loss of dignity. This is tragic to say the least. Many would consider you simply a burden on your family, your friends and society. Not politically correct comments? Sorry the truth rarely is politically correct. You may not want to live "forever" but is this how you would like to spend the last few years of your life?!

Now you say, "I would never live like that, I would end my own life." Well Einstein my answer to you is you don't have a choice! If you put the wrong "oil" in your engine all your life this is where you are likely to end up - on this scrap heap. This is an insidious process. You have long since lost the insight or the ability to have ANY say in the matter. Euthanasia is illegal in most of our societies so no one else is going to risk a jail term trying to "help" you and if they were to ask you if euthanasia is what you desire you just stare blankly back at them. That train left the station years ago so put your views in writing while you still can. Laws may change but my argument is not about euthanasia, not today anyway.

In the example above you are committed to this existence until you die. In the past, you told me it is OK to smoke, be overweight, diabetic or hypertensive and do nothing about your health because it is a free world and "I don't want to live for ever anyway!". Yes, I know, as I have said, I have heard this more than a thousand times. Have you ever thought about how you would like to die? The process of dying may take you 10 years on your current course. Have you ever thought about how much of a burden you want to be on those close to you and on society? You do have a say in this. You can change course now before it is too late.

So, the alternative is you used the right oil in your engine. You are now 70 years of age, bright and full of life. You play golf 3 times per week, belong to multiple clubs and go on long 4WD holidays as you love to explore the outback and go camping. You swim and cycle to keep fit, keeping up with people 20 years your junior. You have 6 grandchildren whom you love spending time with and looking after. You only take a couple of tablets for your blood pressure because your doctor said it was borderline. You are very socially active and you love your life... Do I need to go on? Health span and life span are not the same thing!

I state again this is as much about quality of life as quantity. The metabolic syndrome and all that it codes for and ageing are very closely intertwined. They cannot be easily separated. They come together in the same package. They can both be delayed. Many scientists would now consider the metabolic syndrome a good model for studying premature ageing.

So, the question for those who say, "I don't really want to grow old so I'll do what I like now and suffer the consequences" is really;

Do you want to get old when you are young or do you want to get old when you are old?

It is really your choice but you must make it as early as possible if you want to prevent premature ageing and all the diseases which come with it. This whole concept of "I don't want to get too old" just doesn't cut it! The diseases all come together with the getting old, you just have to decide at what age you want these diseases, including one of the scariest ones of all, dementia. What I would call the demon of the metabolic syndrome or of ageing.

So, one of the ways to avoid ageing and age related diseases and live to your maximal potential age in a good state of physical and mental wellbeing is to "do everything right" in terms of lifestyle including diet and exercise. This may take you to the 90-100 age but much more importantly you will look and feel younger than your stated age and be able to enjoy much more that life has to offer. I will go through the options available to you in subsequent chapters.

The trouble here is we have been giving you a lot of wrong information and advice for the last 60 or 70 years. I hope this book goes part of the way to changing this.

The next step if you are interested is going to be how you go about actually interfering with or blocking the ageing process to exceed your maximal potential age. There are billions or trillions of dollars in potential profits for the drug companies coming to those who can invent and patent a medication as the elixir of life. This is not fantasy or science fiction, we are nearly there. I will explain the metabolic basis of these medications and how they are likely to work later in the book. In the meantime, there are many naturally available compounds and medications which have a modest effect and are available to you now.

CHAPTER 4

The Metabolic syndrome and why you need to avoid it

The metabolic syndrome is to the 21st century what the bubonic plague was to the 14th century. The bubonic plague was an infectious "black death" which swept through Europe and caused the premature death of somewhere between 25 and 60% of the population, death usually occurring within 10 days of infection. The bacteria which caused this is called Yersinia Pestis and is still around today. Now the metabolic syndrome or insulin resistance is not quite as quick but it is just as deadly. The outcome is the same. In its many guises, it accounts for the premature death of about half the population. I'm sure many of you would agree that spending 10 years with dementia and faecal incontinence in a nursing home is probably a much more unpleasant way of dying than with a brief infectious illness. Perhaps you would have been better off living in the 14th century.

This enemy is very sneaky and insidious and may well be on top of you before you even see it coming, like a leopard in the tree above you. This is particularly likely with all the other distractions and stressors our current busy lifestyle has to offer. We don't have time to worry about our health or look up in the trees when walking. Remember rather than ageing causing disease from wear and tear, it may be the diseases which speed up ageing. The metabolic syndrome just happens to be very good at this.

To stay young and healthy you need to avoid getting these diseases in the first place. The first of these is obesity as it is strongly associated with the metabolic syndrome and all that goes with it, including more rapid ageing. There is good evidence the metabolic syndrome is associated with increased all-cause mortality (risk of dying) and with shortened overall lifespan when compared to the general population.

Guize L,Thomas Diabetes Care, 30: 2381–2387, 2007

Zambon S, Diabetes Care, 32:153–159, 2009

The metabolic syndrome is well recognised as being associated with early ageing. We may be the first generation in recent history to have potentially shorter natural lifespans than our parents because of this issue.

Nunn AV,Bell JD,Guy GW (2009) Lifestyle-induced metabolic inflexibility and accelerated ageing syndrome: insulin resistance, friend or foe?. Nutr Metab (Lond.), 6: 16.

So, what is this "metabolic syndrome" and how do you

avoid falling prey to this vile predator who is currently raping and pillaging our society?

The metabolic syndrome is caused largely, by too much energy in, in the way of food and too little out in the way of energy expenditure. Exercise only makes up a small part of the energy out, most of this expenditure just comes simply from staying alive. Sure but, before you say, "it's not my fault, it runs in my family" nothing is that simple, hopefully not even you! (But I have my doubts at times when many of you attempt to use this argument). Let me explain. There have been more than 50 genes identified which predispose you to, or if you like, increase the risk of your developing insulin resistance and all that follows. For you to develop the syndrome and for it to flourish it needs a fertile soil in which it (and you) can grow. That fertile soil we call an "obesogenic environment." It doesn't just "happen", because "my mother was diabetic!" Blaming your mother is the same thing as you are blaming her for your getting sunburnt, "because she gave me fair skin" when really you were the one who made the decision to go out in the sun. The obesogenic environment implies an abundance of high calorie foods and less need for energy expenditure or exercise, such as having a car to drive around in.

Now when we say your genes may predispose you to getting these conditions if exposed to this environment, it is more complex again. The point is the genes involved are not necessarily all yours.

Getting confused? I certainly am! I am not pretending we have all the answers. The genes inside you really are not all yours. There are many more genes in your gut belonging to the bacteria residing there, than there are in you. These bacterial genes outnumber your genes by a factor of 150/1. The genes belonging to the bacteria in your gut are probably more important than your own genes in driving this process of insulin resistance and predisposing you to some of these diseases. These bacteria are very metabolically active and both communicate with you and control you in ways you would not believe possible. We are only just beginning to understand and marvel at this. The bacteria to which these genes belong are influenced by many things such as your diet, how you were born (caesarean section vs natural vaginal delivery), use of antibiotics particularly during your childhood and the cleanliness of your childhood environment. Clean is not necessarily better, yet another piece of bad advice perpetuated by the health profession over the last century.

The metabolic syndrome is not the whole story when it comes to the rate at which we age but it is an important piece of the puzzle and one we can do something about. This process is all about insulin and resistance to the action of insulin termed, "insulin resistance". Every time you eat a large load of carbohydrate, such as sugar or as complex carbohydrates in bread and potatoes for example, this is all absorbed into you blood stream as simple sugars called glucose or fructose. The complex carbohydrates are just long chains of these sugars and the body cuts them into individual links in the gut prior to them passing into the blood and causing a spike in the level of you blood sugar. Now the hormone that controls the level of the sugar in your blood is insulin. When your blood sugar spikes the insulin goes galloping off after it to rein it in, and get it down to an acceptable level which is not toxic to your body. It does this by opening the gates in the cell membranes and letting the glucose go out of the blood stream and into the cells.

The trouble is when you do this over and over and over again, simply by having that "healthy" low fat high carbohydrate breakfast the doctors and dieticians have been telling you is healthy every day, the poor old horse gets tired and cannot keep the galloping up. The cell membrane gates get stiff and will not open as easily to let the glucose into the cells so more and more insulin is required to do the same job. The hinges on those membrane gates are getting rusty. This is the state of insulin resistance. You are now developing the metabolic syndrome, a syndrome in part related to ageing but also a syndrome which in turn causes acceleration of the ageing process.

It is probably reasonable to view this as a state of carbohydrate poisoning or overload out of balance with the rate of use of the carbohydrate through exercise.

Excessive protein probably also plays a role bringing this on earlier as I will explain in later chapters.

The definition of the metabolic syndrome includes 3 of the following:

- High blood fats

- High blood pressure

- Raised blood insulin level relative to the sugar level (insulin resistance)

- Low levels of good cholesterol (HDL)

- Truncal (abdominal) obesity

The diseases which follow the onset of this syndrome include:

- Fatty liver disease, which may progress on to cirrhosis of the liver and liver cancer without a drop of alcohol ever touching your lips. Fatty liver disease is now amongst the commonest reason for needing liver transplantation. Liver cancer is on the rise and rise. The tsunami of liver cancer is just about to hit the shore, it is predicted about 20-30 years after the onset of the fatty liver disease or if you like the onset of the obesity epidemic.

- type 2 diabetes, where the insulin can no longer control the level of the glucose in the blood stream and the glucose level rises. The insulin levels, at least initially, are very high in type 2 diabetes.

- Cardiovascular disease or clogging up of the arteries around your body. This is very important and is the most common cause of death in western society.

If these arteries are in your heart you have a heart attack, if they are running to your brain you have a stroke, if it is the artery to your eye you go blind in that eye. If they are in your leg and cannot be unblocked, we cut your leg off. Black and white, no second chances. There are obviously other factors like smoking which may contribute to vascular disease but the metabolic syndrome does a great job all on its own. It is not clear if the vascular disease is caused primarily by the high blood fats, the high blood sugar, the high blood insulin, the high blood pressure or the more rapid ageing but all these and other factors may contribute. This results in the loss of the smooth Teflon like lining in the arteries so particles in the blood stream begin sticking to the inside lining and eventually block the artery.

- Kidney failure associated with type 2 diabetes, now the commonest cause for needing to be dialysed on an artificial kidney machine or have a kidney transplant. The only alternative is death.

- Up to double the risk of multiple common cancers including breast, bowel, prostate, uterus, cervix, ovary, kidney, oesophagus, gall bladder, liver and pancreas just to mention a few.

- Dementia

- Gout

- Osteoarthritis

- Polycystic ovarian syndrome and infertility

- Sleep Apnoea

I want to say a bit more about cancer here, primarily because it is a scary word and tends to make people sit up in their chairs and listen when I am seeing them in consultation. This in turn is associated with a higher chance they will actually make the lifestyle changes I am suggesting, not just say they will to get me off their case. Obesity and the metabolic syndrome are strongly associated with one another and reducing weight in many cases cures the metabolic syndrome. Obesity per se is associated with an increased risk of developing and dying from many things including cancer, type 2 diabetes and cardiovascular disease. This is likely related in a large part to the associated metabolic syndrome.

A recent review of obesity and cancer risk looked at 204 meta-analyses looking for "strong evidence" for an association between cancer type and obesity. They looked at 36 types of cancer and found this strong evidence of association for 11 cancers which are predominantly cancers associated with the gut or with being a woman. These cancers are of the lower oesophagus or gullet, the upper stomach, bile ducts and gall bladder, pancreas, and the colon and rectum in the gut. In women, the risk of cancers of the breast, ovary and uterus are markedly increased with a steady increase for each increment in increased weight. Kidney cancer and multiple myeloma (blood) cancer are also strongly associated with weight. There were multiple other cancers associated with weight but the evidence linking them was not as strong so I will leave these out. The problem is the worldwide prevalence of obesity has tripled in men and more than doubled in women in the last 4 decades taking the number from 857 million in 1980 to 2.1 billion in 2013 and the increase shows no sign of abating. If you look at something like breast cancer (post menopause), obesity roughly doubles your risk for this. Weight loss to prevent this is likely to be very much more effective than screening with mammography in preventing breast cancer related death. It just doesn't seem to be politically correct to say this. Sorry I'm not politically correct. I just state the facts.

This is not a complete list of diseases associated with the metabolic syndrome and new additions are a regular occurrence. These diseases share one thing in common. They are much more likely if you are in a state of insulin resistance and they are associated with an acceleration of the ageing process. It is not clear to us what drives many of the diseases but the high insulin level I believe is part of the process, not necessarily the high blood sugar. You need some insulin to keep you alive but it is toxic at high levels and may well shorten your life. This is likely related to mTOR activation discussed in the next chapter. Literally too much of a good thing.

The important point here for you as an individual is this high level of insulin is likely a lifestyle choice. Your lifestyle choice. It is not a given. It is not your parents fault. It is something you can do a lot about. Primarily with careful dietary choices and exercise as discussed in the prior publication "Death by Carbs". Get off your arse and make the right choices! I would much rather you did this than have to diagnose your bowel cancer for you in 10 years' time. I already diagnose multiple cancers every week and I'm getting sick of this as they are often unnecessary cancers. Many didn't have to happen.

CHAPTER 5

The Mechanistic Target of Rapamycin (m-TOR) The Grand Conductor.

The central processing unit (CPU) for growth and metabolism

Well I know this one sounds like Latin but it is a key modulator of ageing and age related disease and we cannot have this discussion without paying some attention to it. I am going to get a bit technical in this discussion and it is not crucial you understand it or read this chapter but I think it is fascinating, so if you are interested, try to stay with me. It will make it easier for you to understand the mechanisms by which some diets, exercise and medications or supplements work in possibly delaying the ageing process. If you are a medical practitioner this section is compulsory.

There has been a staggering amount of research into this and I am going to give you a bit of an overview into the history and where it all began.

This started in the 1970s when a compound with promise as a new antifungal agent was discovered in the soil of a Polynesian island. This compound was called rapamycin and the bacteria in the soil which produces it is called Streptomyces hygroscopicus. The rapamycin was then found to impair cellular division and found useful in immunosuppression, impairing rejection of a transplanted kidney or liver and in preventing blockage of coronary artery stents. Interestingly it was noted that the kidney transplant patients who were treated with rapamycin (also called Sirolimus) got far fewer skin cancers than those treated with other immunosuppressant drugs. When it was also discovered to prolong the life expectancy of yeasts, worms, fruit flies and mice things got really interesting. Perhaps it would have this effect on people?

The search was then on to determine how the compound actually worked in these organisms to achieve its life prolonging effects.

The enzymes complexes, or more correctly called protein kinases, on which this compound works, were called the mechanistic Target of Rapamycin. There were 2 main complexes discovered, labelled imaginatively as mTOR1 and mTOR2. Further assessment of these complexes showed that they are crucial for life. They are inside all cells and over hundreds of millions of years of evolution they have hardly changed, from single cellular yeasts, to worms to fruit flies to humans. It seems that if you tried to alter them too much in evolution you ended up as one of those fossils in a rock and did not pass your genes on to anything living on the planet today. They must be important.

It also became apparent that these enzyme complexes were the true grand conductors of ageing, growth and of metabolism inside the cell. We are only just beginning to sort out the mechanisms of how they do this and the more we look the more interesting it becomes.

mTOR is far from a simple switch which you can turn on or off. It is more like an intracellular computer which can cope with multiple inputs, process them, and then put out multiple messages controlling numerous downstream events which include the rate of ageing, growth and metabolism. It is complex and unlike male human beings whom we know can only do one thing at a time, mTOR can communicate with many messengers bringing in information, giving multiple instructions down the line to others all at the same time. A bit like a woman?

Some of these instructions relate to cellular growth and production of protein which allows for organisms to grow, for cells to divide, muscles to grow and for the species to reproduce and survive. This protein allows for wounds to heal. You can only build those muscles or produce new offspring or heal those wounds if you have the resources with which to do so — the basic building blocks and the energy to put them together.

For this reason, the mTOR is a bit like the foreman on a building site who gives the OK to the other workmen to start building your house when the bricks and the cement arrive. You cannot build a brick wall without bricks and cement or the energy (workmen) to put this together. You cannot build protein without its building blocks which we call amino acids, and without energy to put them together. These amino acids and energy levels are some of the many critical things that the mTOR senses before it gives instructions to start assembling them into the amino acid chains we call proteins. This makes sense for survival of a species. If there is no food available the organism stops growing and goes into a state of relative hibernation thus using far less of its resources. Once the dry season is over and the rains arrive food is plentiful again and the organism can grow and reproduce once more. mTOR is then switched ON when those rains arrive and food and resources are plentiful — at a cellular level. If cells had no control over their cellular metabolism to allow them to use resources wisely and not run out, they would die very quickly. This would be a bit like a bush fire, out of control and when all the resources are consumed the fire goes out, or the cell dies. Single cells need a constant supply of energy to survive. This is how cyanide works — it blocks energy production in a cell and these cells, and the whole organism die in seconds, just like in the movies. A bit like water bombing a fire.

Unfortunately, this process of cellular division and growth is also associated with ageing and death. Once the organism has produced it's off spring the continued stimulation of mTOR while helpful in some respects brings on many diseases and speeds up the ageing process. As discussed earlier, there may only be a limited number of times those cells in your body can divide before you die. Once you get to that magical number of cell divisions your time is up.

At this time of your life - after having your family - you want to drive mTOR very slowly, you need it to keep moving - and you alive - but not going too fast. It is a bit like the accelerator in a car where you only have one tank of petrol to go through the rest of your life with. You can push the pedal to the metal and drive very fast, head held high thumbing your nose and flexing your biceps at the slower drivers and you run out of fuel at 60 miles/years and that is when you die. Alternatively, if you drive slowly and economically you might just get to 120 miles/years before your petrol tank is empty and your time is up.

If you switch mTOR on fully then you are likely to age more rapidly and you seem to develop all the diseases listed in the section on the metabolic syndrome. You are likely to die younger. It does not seem to matter if you are a single cellular yeast, a worm, a fruit fly or a mouse. I am extrapolating a bit here to include humans but in my opinion you are not much different from a mouse or a rat and the same rules apply in life and in death. The mTOR molecule is almost identical and that is what we are talking about.

If you inhibit the mTOR in all these animal models with rapamycin the animals live longer. We haven't experimented on humans yet but your time is coming. We just have to find safer drugs to use than rapamycin because of the side effects and we don't have any idea what dose to use. These side effects include raised blood fats, diabetes, mouth ulcers and predisposition to viral and fungal infections. Your immune system cells need to be able to divide to protect you. No point in dying young from a simple infection. Unfortunately, when used long term in humans rapamycin inhibits mTOR2 which is important for insulin sensitivity, resulting in diabetes. We think we only want to inhibit the mTOR1 complex and if we could do this we would protect you from diabetes. We just need more specific drugs.

There is a safer drug which has been used for more than 60 years to treat diabetes and it is also very cheap, unlike the new anti-ageing drugs which are on the horizon. It inhibits mTOR1 only and diabetics treated with this have been shown to live longer, and get less heart disease, cancer and dementia than those treated with alternatives. I will discuss this in later chapters.

So, if you do not want to stimulate mTOR 1 later in

life what are the things you need to avoid unnecessary stimulation? Well this is what the book is about and is discussed in more detail in subsequent chapters. Remember the downside of inhibiting mTOR 1 is reduced muscle growth and this may be an issue in the elderly who need muscle strength to remain mobile and independent. It is also a negative if you are in a body building competition or in the Olympics, as your muscles may not grow as large or as strong. I think the positives outweigh the negatives here however, particularly with respect to your most important organ, your brain.

Your brain cells do very little if any division once you are an adult. It is generally a downhill ride or slide with loss of brain cells and brain cell function throughout your adult life. To some extent when you inhibit mTOR this process stops or slows. With the slowing of metabolism your brain has time to do some spring cleaning around its cells. The cell's vacuum cleaner – lysosymes - clean up all the litter that has been left lying around when these cells were very busy and didn't have time to clean. This litter includes protein complexes which when they accumulate can clump together and interfere with brain cell functioning and potentially predispose you to diseases such as Alzheimer's disease. These protein complexes or plaques are called beta-amyloid and they are numerous in Alzheimer's disease.

This process of cleaning them up and getting rid of

them is called autophagy.

Autophagy is a very important process described below. It is the recycling system in your cells. Just like you cannot fill a planet up with rubbish and expect to keep living there unaffected, you cannot fill your cells up with rubbish and expect them to keep functioning properly. Autophagy allows for your cells to perform orderly degradation of the intracellular rubbish, or cellular components which no longer have a use, and recycle them into useful components again. To clean up the mess. This process produces energy to keep cell alive in times of cellular starvation or stress.

m-TOR and Dementia/Alzheimer's disease

If I had to tell you what I find the scariest part of ageing it is the risk of becoming demented and a burden on others. Cancer scares me less because at least you are not going to be around burdening others for too long. Cognitive decline can be shown in normal people on testing from the age of 45 onwards. I cannot prove to you that if you take drugs to block m-TOR you will not get dementia or that they definitely work in people. The trouble is by the time this has been proven it may well be too late for you to act. It is unlikely you can reverse the process of dementia, it is more a question of stopping it happening in the first place. So, what evidence do we have? Well the evidence is in mice, which are not people but they are not that dissimilar in the things that happen with age. The evidence in mice is described as "striking"

The first thing you tend to notice as mice (or people) age is loss of spatial learning and memory. Spatial learning for you essentially means remembering the way to an address you have driven to before on the other side of the city. In the mice in this study this meant finding something in a maze, after repetitive training showing them where the treat was. 2-month-old mice learn this very much more quickly than 18-month-old (middle aged) mice and this was well shown. When you treat the 18-month-old mice with rapamycin from the age of 2 months they learn new tasks very much more quickly than mice not treated. The age dependent cognitive deficit is prevented. (p <0.0001, showing this is highly statistically significant) The researchers could also show that mTOR signalling was reduced as were pro-inflammatory cytokines or damaging messengers in the brain. These increased normally with age in untreated, compared to treated mice.

Ageing Cell (2012) 11, pp326-335, Lifelong rapamycin administration ameliorates age dependent cognitive deficits by reducing IL-1B and enhancing NMDA signalling Smita Majumder et al.

In another study of mice fed rapamycin this was shown to extend lifespan and, "enhance the cognitive function in young adult mice and block age-associated cognitive decline in older animals. In addition, mice fed with rapamycin supplemented chow showed decreased anxiety and depressive like behaviour at all ages tested"

Neuroscience. Volume 223, 25 October 2012, Pages 102–113 Chronic inhibition of mammalian target of rapamycin by rapamycin modulates cogntive and non-cognitive components of behaviour throughout lifespan in mice J. Halloran

These studies speak for themselves. Blocking mTOR achieves miracles in blocking age related cognitive decline, at least in mice!

mTOR and cancer

I cannot prove to you that mTOR is the cause of cancer, partly because this would be incorrect and a gross oversimplification. What we can do however is look at what happens when we inhibit the enzyme complex mTOR and we have just the drug to do this, yes you guessed it rapamycin.

The first group in whom this effect was observed were patients undergoing kidney transplantation. This group are at markedly increased risk for cancer, particularly skin cancers presumably because the immunosuppression they require to stop them from rejecting their new kidney also stops their immune system from rejecting early cancers which may develop.

Rapamycin inhibits the growth of many cells. This inhibition of the immune cell's division (T and B cell lymphocytes) is thought to account for rapamycin's immune inhibition effect which prevents rejection of organ transplants. It is also felt to inhibit the cellular growth and division in new cancers. In numerous studies looking at kidney transplant recipients, those who received rapamycin had roughly half the number of skin cancers when compared to those receiving other immunosuppressant drugs. This has been shown in numerous studies. Studies also show that other types of cancers are less likely in rapamycin treated patients when compared to patients treated with standard immunosuppressant drugs, including lung, throat, larynx, kidney, bowel, stomach, prostate, breast cancer and others.

J Am Soc Nephrol. 2006 Feb;17(2):581-9

mTOR is very important in cellular growth and proliferation, as has been discussed. The cells that grow the fastest are cancer cells and it is reasonable to assume that the loss of control of growth here may partly relate to turbocharging of the mTOR enzyme complex in these cancer cells. This is indeed the case with mTOR which is up regulated in almost all human cancers, allowing for rapid uncontrolled growth and cellular division. A bit like a turbocharged car out of control with the accelerator stuck down to the floor. It is not surprising then that inhibiting mTOR has then been shown to reduce the incidence of cancer in groups at high risk such as kidney transplant patients, despite their being immunosuppressed where you would be expecting a higher, not lower, cancer incidence.

It follows then that mTOR inhibitors may be very useful in treating cancers and they were initially tested with great enthusiasm hoping we had found a cancer cure. As is often the case in medicine things were more complicated than we first thought and although they do have some efficacy in fighting cancer they were not a universal cure. They also came at some cost in terms of side effects. A good deal of hope remains however and many groups are working on making new drugs based on this mechanism for use in cancer, drugs that are more specific in their targeting. Drugs which are more like a rifle than a shot gun, as rapamycin is best regarded.

mTOR and Ageing

This enzyme complex is right at the centre when it comes to controlling the rate of cellular ageing. This control is an important protection mechanism for the survival of a species. Remember the things that switch mTOR on are essentially food such as glucose and amino acids, or the hormones which are secreted in response to protein or carbohydrate, insulin like growth factors and insulin. Switching mTOR on allows the organism to grow and to reproduce, which it does when food is plentiful.

Switching mTOR off allows the species to stay alive when food and resources are not plentiful so that when the dry spell ends you are still there to be able to breed and reproduce. If this was not possible climate events such as droughts would result in much higher levels of extinction of life.

Evolution has shaped mTOR to do this over hundreds of millions of years. Evolution does not care what happens after reproduction, it is simply a mathematical equation dictating the probability of survival of a species. Individuals and their life span are meaningless to evolution as long as the species as a whole survives. Mathematical equations of probability do not have feelings, they are just used as tools to explain why things happen. After reproduction, the sooner you are discarded the better unless your short-term survival benefits the survival of the species as discussed in an earlier chapter.

You should look at mTOR as a tool you can manipulate to promote a longer healthy lifespan or health span if you prefer this term. You are trying to trick mTOR into believing you are in a fasting state. That you are living during at time of drought or famine. A lot of this book discusses the ways we can manipulate mTOR to our advantage and provides some of the evidence for various approaches. The lists below are far from complete, they are to give you a general understanding of mTOR function.

We all, including the scientists are at the tip of the ice berg of knowledge here and have a lot to learn.

If you switch mTOR ON you get:

(1) More rapid ageing with a shorter lifespan

(2) Earlier onset of multiple diseases which are associated with ageing including but not limited to;

- Type 2 diabetes

- Cardiovascular disease (heart attacks and strokes)

- Osteoarthritis

- Gout

- Multiple common cancers

- Dementia

- Muscle growth

- Fat growth

These "diseases" result in a reduced health span as well as lifespan. At what age would you like to get these diseases?

If you switch mTOR OFF with a reduction in stimulators or the use of inhibitors you get:

- Reduced incidence of all the diseases listed above with prolongation of life span and health span.

- Reduced muscle growth and presumably muscle strength and exercise capability but this may not be very significant to your lifestyle unless you do highly competitive sport, weight lifting or your job requires a lot of physical strength. Muscles are also important in the elderly however for mobility.

- Reduced wound healing (theoretically)

- Reduced fertility (a woman's menstrual cycle stops with fasting long enough)

- Reduced rate of growth if you are still growing (and I mean for those of you growing upwards and those of you growing outwards!)

- Autophagy. Remember this is critically important in promoting longevity. It is the major pathway by which your cells clean up all the mess in terms of intracellular organelles and large molecules which are littering your cells and interfering with their full functioning. This is essential for recycling your resources such as amino acids during periods of starvation. Your cells switch into a repair and maintenance mode. This is a specific mTOR 1 inhibition effect and probably explains many of the beneficial effects of mTOR 1 inhibitors, particularly in the discussion of dementia above.

So, you see it is not all good or all bad, no matter what path you chose. If you are in a hospital bed recovering from a motor car accident with multiple trauma, or you are trying to have a family you do not want to switch mTOR off completely. If you are trying to win a weight lifting competition you are not going to do so unless you switch your mTOR on, but remember this will come at a cost and nothing in life is free! Everything is a balance.

I don't think it matters what you do in the short term so don't panic and change your behaviour immediately, at least finish the book! Once you are moving into middle age and have had your children however I think you need to start erring on the side of caution in the long term and avoiding over stimulation of mTOR.

What stimulates mTOR?

- Amino acids particularly branched chain amino acids such leucine, isoleucine and valine, found in larger proportions in animal protein than plant protein. These amino acids are also essential for life. They are the building blocks of protein. They are the strongest mTOR stimulators.

- Glucose; blood sugar

- Insulin, a peptide (short protein) hormone in the blood stream which controls the levels of blood sugar or glucose by moving the glucose out of the blood stream into cells where it can be used for energy.

- Insulin like growth factors (IGF). IGF-1 is a peptide hormone like insulin, produced in the liver in response to stimulation from growth hormone (released from the pituitary gland in the brain). IGF-1 level is increased by increased dietary protein intake. Many other factors also have an influence on levels to a lesser extent. It works to stimulate growth in tissues through stimulation of mTOR. It is to protein a bit like insulin is to sugar or glucose.

- Oxygen

What are some common inhibitors of mTOR?

- Fasting (with reduction in available glucose and amino acids)

- Exercise

- Rapamycin from which the enzyme complex takes its name. The trouble with rapamycin is we only want to inhibit mTOR 1 and it inhibits 1 and 2. It also has side effects discussed in subsequent chapters.

- Metformin, this is an amazing drug I will discuss in the section on medication options

- Aspirin

- Caffeine

- Resveratrol the pigment in red wine

- Other plant related pigments predominantly in blue and red vegetables or fruits.

- Curcumin (the pigment in turmeric)

- Green tea extract...and many others

The implications of manipulating mTOR are profound at least theoretically in terms of disease and life expectancy. The above inhibitors tend to block the effect of, or activation of, the mTOR complex.

To summarise, switching this mTOR complex on puts your body in the mode of growth, strength and reproduction, necessary for survival of the species. Switching it off puts you in the mode of repair and maintenance so it lasts longer and functions better. This is necessary for your long term healthy survival. It's your choice.

Remember what you put in the top of an equation, or even a simple food processor, determines what comes out the bottom so let me try to show you diagrammatically what I mean. Sorry about the complexity. Look at the input at the top of each of the diagrams and the output at the bottom. It may look a bit complicated but the truly complex part of the diagrams is mTOR. The structure and function of mTOR, and all the feedback loops in this "computer", and its componentry. I've left these things out completely. So, this is a bit of an oversimplification – despite its complexity - but hopefully will convey the message.

Again, the inputs are your lifestyle choices, the outputs simply follow. Compare the input and output sections of the diagrams.

Remember also, in balanced equations, input always equals output.

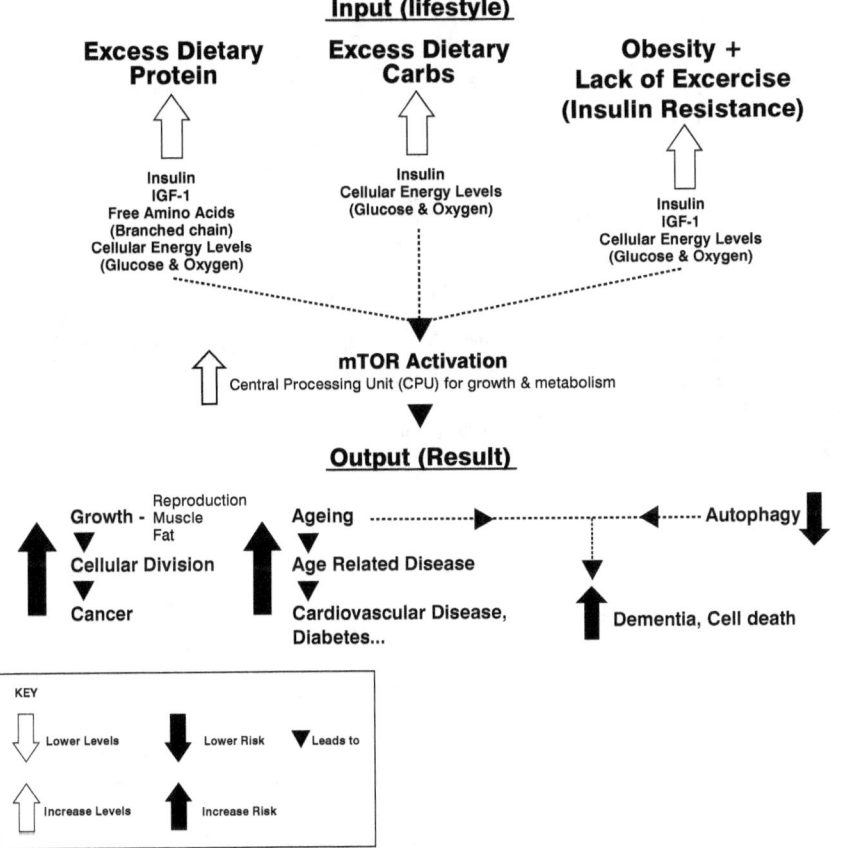

Switching mTOR ON

Input (lifestyle)

Excess Dietary Protein

Insulin
IGF-1
Free Amino Acids
(Branched chain)
Cellular Energy Levels
(Glucose & Oxygen)

Excess Dietary Carbs

Insulin
Cellular Energy Levels
(Glucose & Oxygen)

Obesity + Lack of Excercise (Insulin Resistance)

Insulin
IGF-1
Cellular Energy Levels
(Glucose & Oxygen)

mTOR Activation
Central Processing Unit (CPU) for growth & metabolism

Output (Result)

Growth - Reproduction
Muscle
Fat

Cellular Division

Cancer

Ageing

Age Related Disease

Cardiovascular Disease, Diabetes...

Autophagy

Dementia, Cell death

KEY

Lower Levels

Increase Levels

Lower Risk

Increase Risk

Leads to

Switching mTOR OFF

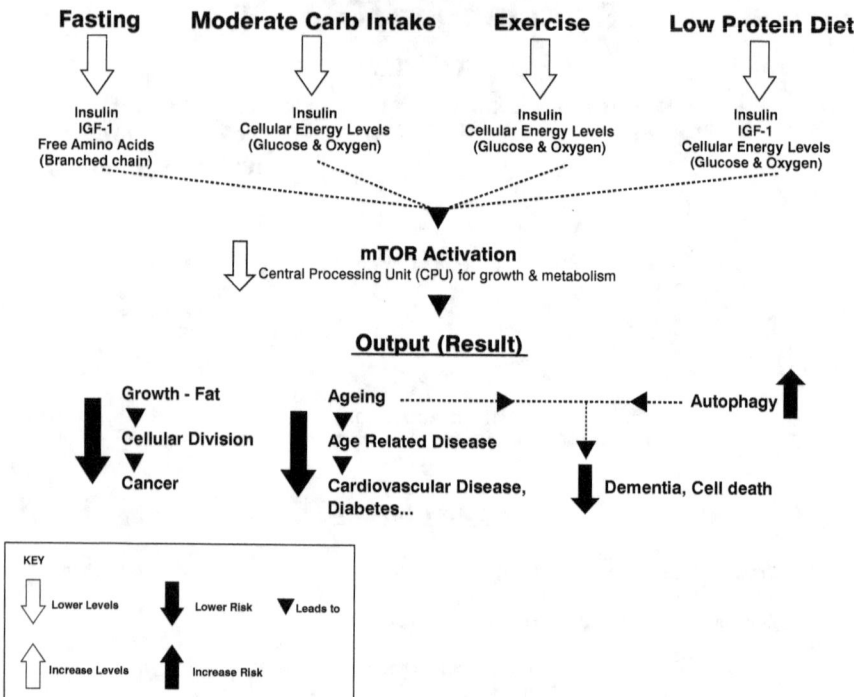

Input (lifestyle)

Fasting **Moderate Carb Intake** **Exercise** **Low Protein Diet**

Insulin
IGF-1
Free Amino Acids
(Branched chain)

Insulin
Cellular Energy Levels
(Glucose & Oxygen)

Insulin
Cellular Energy Levels
(Glucose & Oxygen)

Insulin
IGF-1
Cellular Energy Levels
(Glucose & Oxygen)

mTOR Activation
Central Processing Unit (CPU) for growth & metabolism

Output (Result)

Growth - Fat

Cellular Division

Cancer

Ageing ┈┈┈> Autophagy

Age Related Disease

Cardiovascular Disease,
Diabetes...

Dementia, Cell death

KEY

⇩ Lower Levels   ⬇ Lower Risk   ▼ Leads to

⇧ Increase Levels   ⬆ Increase Risk

63

CHAPTER 6

Sirtuins, PARPs and NAD+

A gain, this chapter is optional and may only be of interest to those of you who have been researching the literature on ageing, and to medical practitioners. If you start yawning skip the chapter. It is very interesting however – possibly the most exciting bit of the book - and is another arm of the ageing process which lends itself to intervention with drugs or natural products to potentially alter the rate at which we age. This arm of the ageing process goes one step further than the mTOR pathways in that these enzymes are responsible for many other processes including repair of DNA which offers the theoretical potential to reverse ageing after it has occurred, albeit to a limited extent. The other exciting thing about the drugs which may activate this system is that they are already here. The downside is they have not been tested properly in humans so taking them is done at a potential risk – we don't know how safe they are to take long term or if they work in humans. Nor do we know what dose to take.

Now I am going to get a bit involved in the biochemistry. These Sirtuins are not completely separable from the mTOR pathways and in part act by facilitating the blocking of mTOR. In mammals, there are 7 of these enzymes or chemicals labelled SIRT1-7. The magnificent seven.

Chemically, Sirtuins are defined as NAD+ dependent deacylases. They are all activated by NAD+. They respond to changes in cellular energy levels, cellular stress and DNA damage and act by switching on genes in the DNA of the cell. These genes enhance the energy efficiency of the cell by switching on its small power plants called mitochondria which use oxygen to burn products and produce energy, resupplying the cells energy reserves by increasing its ATP levels. ATP or adenosine triphosphate is the energy supply in the cell, like the electricity supply in a battery. When the ATP gives up its energy it becomes AMP or adenosine monophosphate. The ratio of ATP to AMP tells you how well charged the cells batteries are. In other words, if there is very little ATP and a lot of AMP you are about to have a power blackout.

AMP activated protein kinase or AMPK is the sensing gauge for this ATP/AMP ratio or battery storage level and senses other possible fuels such as glucose it can use to burn in those mitochondria to make more ATP, or if you like to recharge the cell's batteries. AMPK is switched on when the ATP/AMP or power level in the cell is low. When you switch on AMPK it acts to shut down mTOR and thus conserve energy levels in the cell, saying essentially "we are about to run out of power, shut down everything that is not essential", such as protein assembly (muscle growth, cellular division). In other words, activation of AMPK serves to inhibit mTOR, and to turn ON energy production in the mitochondria. This is the association between the Sirtuins and mTOR as SIRT1 also acts to turn on AMPK thereby inhibiting mTOR with all those desired effects described in the previous chapter. Natural products like resveratrol (pigment in red wine and purple vegetables/fruits) stimulate the activity of SIRT1 which in turn activates AMPK with subsequent inhibition of mTOR. This may be the pathway of action of some of the natural products.

That is probably about as much as we know about how these enzyme complexes, the Sirtuins and mTOR, are linked. There may be many more links it is just that we have not yet uncovered them.

NAD+ (Nicotinamide adenine dinucleotide) is the oxidised form of NADH. You are alive because your body can do controlled reactions transferring electrons and hydrogen atoms. These oxidative or reductive metabolic reactions are the basis of life. These NAD+/NADH molecules are like the oil allowing the gear cogs of these chemical reactions to occur. These little molecules are essential for life, lubricating the reactions by providing electrons or hydrogen atoms. They are described as coenzymes for these reactions which they lubricate, but they also participate in the reaction and are consumed by the reaction, for example, turning NAD+ into NADH.

NAD+ is necessary to activate the Sirtuins. It is probably a thousand times more potent than resveratrol at doing this. As these Sirtuins facilitate DNA repair one would expect them to result in life extension in animal models and indeed this is the case. Their activation has been shown to prolong the life expectancy of yeast, worms, fruit flies and mice. They also prevent disease in these animal models including mouse models of type 2 diabetes, cancer, cardiovascular disease, Parkinson's disease, Alzheimer's disease and inflammatory (autoimmune) disease.

The seven mammalian Sirtuins are a relatively recent discovery and we are again only at the tip of the iceberg in terms of starting to sort out exactly what they all do. Some are found in the nucleus of the cell, some in the cytoplasm and others in the mitochondria. In these positions, they are able to potentially control metabolism – effecting obesity, insulin resistance and diabetes, and to repair damaged DNA reducing the risk of cancer and the rate of ageing. All of which they have been shown to do in mouse models. SIRT1 also seems very important in regulating melatonin and the circadian rhythm or body clock which also has implications in the metabolic syndrome and ageing.

The exciting thing about these wonder enzymes is

that their activity can be stimulated relatively simply by a small molecule, NAD+. NAD+ levels have been shown to decline gradually with age and in association with this decline the activity of SIRT follows suit, gradually declining, with a subsequent increase in all the age-related diseases we have discussed. Declining NAD+ and SIRT1 levels with ageing seem to interfere with communication between the cell's control centre, the nucleus, and its power stations the mitochondria. This results in loss of mitochondrial function with ageing and loss of cellular functions needing energy. These chemicals also seem to be important for communication between your brains appetite centre, the hypothalamus, and your body's fat reserves, with a subsequently increase in the size of your fat reserves as you age. The hypothalamus also seems to be important for ageing at a whole-body level. Preventing this decline in the NAD+ and SERT1 levels with aging, potentially prevents the aging, at least in mice.

It follows then that if you give NAD+, which is made from vitamin B3, and comes in several other forms such as nicotinamide or nicotinic acid, you will potentially prevent ageing in people. NAD supplementation studies in 2009 unfortunately did not live up to this hope. NAD is too big a molecule to get through cellular membranes and into cells.

Shin-ichiro Imai et al, 2009 Cell Biochem Biophys.

When one gives the NAD+ as a precursor called

nicotinamide mononucleotide (NMN), which can be taken by mouth and is converted in the cell into NAD+ it does indeed live up to its expectations. NMN is a smaller molecule which can get through the cell membrane into the cell. If you combine two NMN molecules your basically get one NAD+. This potentially has huge implications for humans but at the time of printing beneficial effect has only been demonstrated in mice.

In a very recent study over 12 months' mice were fed NMN or placebo in their drinking water. There was no apparent toxicity in the NMN fed mice and its supplementation resulted in prevention of normal age-associated decline in many physiological areas.

These included: -Suppression of age associated weight gain, despite higher food intake

- Enhanced energy metabolism and mitochondrial function, even when sleeping, predominantly from fat burning, not glucose.

- Promotion of physical activity

- Improved insulin sensitivity

- Improved lipid profile (lower cholesterol and triglycerides)

- Improved eyesight, with effects on cones and rods (colour and black/white vision)

- Reduction in activation of age related genes

- Improved bone and muscle strength

- Improved immune function.

In summary, the results were "too good to be true". It seemed to prevent ageing and age related disease with no side effects, or at least none the mice complained of. The NMN was well absorbed into the blood stream and converted in the cells to NAD+. Numerous other studies on NMN in mice, and of another precursor of NAD+, Nicotinamide riboside (NR), have shown similar effects in mouse models including prevention of Alzheimer's disease, noise induced hearing loss, cardiovascular disease, cancer and obesity.

Long-term Administration of Nicotinamide Mononucleotide Mitigates Age-Associated Physiological decline in Mice. Mills et al, Dec 2016.

Let us look at another article, again published in 2016, which looks at vascular disease, or disease of the arteries in mice as they age. Mice as I keep suggesting are not really that different to humans and both species have similar age related changes in the artery cell walls with increasing age. What happens is your arteries lose compliance or stretch ability. They change from being like expansile rubber tubes to rigid steel like pipes. As the old artery cannot expand to take the blood ejected from the heart, the pressure in the tube (blood pressure) rises and the pulse wave moves very much more quickly down the rigid old pipe than it would down a young rubbery tube. This pulse wave velocity can be used to measure large elastic artery stiffness and rises in the pulse wave velocity are a very good predictor of vascular disease, for example the likelihood of you having a stroke or a heart attack in the near future. In this study, the researchers took old and young mice and compared them. The young mice had a lot of elastin or rubber like material in their largest artery (the aorta) and the old mice had a lot of steel like material called type 1 collagen in their aortas at base line as was expected.

A group of old mice were then given NMN in their drinking water for 8 weeks at a target dose of 300mg per kg per day. The amazing finding was that the NMN treated mice had their large elastic type arteries transformed back to being indistinguishable from those of the young mice. In other word the stiffness of their arteries became the same as the young mice again, completely reversing the effects of ageing. The levels of collagen 1 and elastin were restored to the levels of the young mice as was the pulse wave velocity. The levels of NAD+ were increased 3 times in the arteries of the treated old mice and their SIRT-1 levels increase to be equal to those of the young mice with the NMN supplementation. The treatment also reduced the oxidative stress in the arteries of the old mice which is also important in age related arterial dysfunction. Amazing stuff!

Nicotinamide mononucleotide supplementation reverses vascular dysfunction and oxidative stress with ageing in mice. Ageing Cell. Jun 2016, Picciotto et al

Nicotinamide riboside (NR) is another precursor to NAD+ and is probably at least as good or better at raising the levels of NAD+ in the cells. Studies have been done with this in mice showing that it protects the animals from animal models of dementia improving cognitive function and improving the levels of NAD+ in the brain. This effect is associated with a reduction in the waste proteins found in brain cells of mouse models of Alzheimer's disease. Other studies of NR have shown similar effects to NMN with protection of mice fed a high fat diet from obesity and from diabetes. A single dose of NR will normalise insulin sensitivity, albeit transiently, in a diabetic mouse.

Canto et al, Cell Metabolism; 2012, 838-47.

These NAD+ effects may not all relate to Sirtuins. There are other enzymes which depend on and are also activated by NAD+ and these include PARPs (Poly ADP-ribose polymerase). Sorry about the names. This family of proteins is found in the nucleus of the cell. Its primary function is repair of damaged DNA but a subset of these proteins is also associated with repair of telomeres and we know how important these may be. The levels of these proteins in the cell nucleus seems to be associated with life expectancy. For example, the levels are much higher in people who live over 100 when compared to people who die at 70 years of age. The levels also correlate with the lifespan difference between species. For example, the levels in humans are 5 times higher than they are in rats, suggesting PARP mediated DNA repair capability contributes to mammalian longevity. This is true of all mammalian species tested. PARP levels predict life expectancy of the species. You want to keep these enzymes active also and to do this you need to keep your NAD+ levels up. PARP activity also declines with the age associated reduction in NAD+ levels, with resultant accelerated accumulation of unrepaired DNA damage as you age.

So where do I get this wonder drug? I hear your say. Well there are natural vegetable sources such as edamame (immature soybeans), broccoli, cucumber (seed and peel), cabbage, and fruits such as avocado and tomato. Mushrooms also contain variable amounts. These foods contain between 0-2 mg per 100g. The mice were fed 100-300mg/Kg/day. To put that in other terms, if you weigh 75kg and the broccoli you are eating is 1mg per 100g or 10mg per kg, you would need to eat 300/10 x 75 (2250kg) of broccoli in a day to get the dose the highest dosed mice got. That is greater than 2 tonnes of broccoli per day. I know some of you can eat a lot but this is pushing it a little bit. When your mother said, "eat your greens Johnnie" I don't think this is what she intended.

The good news is that both NMN and NR are commercially available in more concentrated forms. The bad news is it is difficult to know the quality of the products you buy. As this is a relatively new area with demand outstripping supply, there will be a lot of sharks out there substituting and selling substandard quality medication, which may not even be what they say it is. Worse still their formulation may be toxic.

The second "bad news" bit is I have been talking about mice. This is not Metformin which we have been experimenting with in other people for 70 years just to make sure it is safe for you to take. There is as yet no data on either safety or efficacy in humans. That said, this is pretty exciting stuff! There will be data soon. It is expensive so perhaps until we have that data you should eat your broccoli and buy shares in the company which makes these products.

CHAPTER 7

Diet

Diet is arguably the most important thing we are going to discuss here and as I have eluded to in the introduction I think we have been going about this all the wrong way. The guidelines for a healthy diet are seriously flawed in my opinion and I will endeavour to explain to you why I believe this to be the case and what I think you should be doing with your diet. Look at the people around you, does it look like doctors and other health professionals have been giving the right advice? What has been the result of this "right advice?" Remember always there will be many "experts" who disagree with me and will be vocal about doing so.

Carbohydrate

Now I know many of you feel I have an issue with carbohydrate and this is certainly the case when one looks at society with the incidence of obesity and type

2 diabetes skyrocketing. In Australia, we are already amongst the fattest people on earth, with 2/3 of us falling into the range of obese or overweight based on BMI calculation. In this majority of our population who, generally speaking, tend to be insulin resistant, this issue of carbohydrate intake really does matter.

By insulin resistant I mean they require much higher blood levels of insulin to achieve the same blood glucose level when compared to a thin and generally insulin sensitive person. There are always exceptions to these rules because there are other factors at play which determine the level of insulin resistance, including your genetic makeup, the type of bugs in your bowel and perhaps how much protein you have consumed in your life.

The problem with being insulin resistant is that you need persistently high levels of insulin in your body for the insulin to do its work and when it comes to ageing, insulin is not your friend. Again, speaking generally, insulin levels tend to parallel weight gain. The bigger you get the more insulin resistant you become and consequently the higher the insulin levels needed to keep your blood sugar levels under control.

This is a double-edged sword. Once you have a lot of fat on board with high insulin levels it gets very hard to lose weight. This is the reason weight gain seems to be such a one-way street for many people.

Insulin is the enemy to weight loss. It is best regarded

as a large padlock on the back shed where you store all your body fat. It blocks everything to do with getting rid of the fat. It blocks you getting into the shed, it blocks you mobilising any fat or taking it out of the shed, and if you were lucky enough to get any out into the blood stream it blocks you using or burning the fat. The blood level of fats (triglyceride) just stay high. The body is switched – or should I say forced - into a mode of burning carbohydrate only and I mean ONLY. Insulin is a very powerful hormone and if it says NO to burning or mobilising fat reserves there is no option for negotiation. The fat on your hips and abdomen stays right where it is. The situation is hopeless, the game is lost – and I am sure that is just how many of you feel. It does not matter how much you exercise or how hard you try to diet, nothing seems to work.

That is unless you go back to basics and think. We must get insulin levels down to lose weight (fat).

What stimulates insulin release to keep it high? No prizes for this one. It is carbohydrate and it is everywhere in your diet if you are eating a typical modern western diet. If you are not sure where or what carbohydrate is you need to read prior publications such as "Death by Carbs" which will make it abundantly clear for you.

So, the answer to losing weight and dramatically dropping your insulin levels is a low carbohydrate and preferably low to moderate protein diet, as protein also causes insulin release raising its levels.

If you fail to get the high insulin levels down you will proceed along your merry way to getting diabetes, heart and other vascular disease, numerous potential cancers and dementia. They are all just waiting for you. A bit like stops on a one-way train trip you have just commenced with the last stop being your death. You will get to the last stop at a younger age because the metabolic syndrome you are developing is a turbo charged form of ageing, both old age and disease come more quickly. The evidence that people with the metabolic syndrome, and all that goes with it, die younger is black and white. It's a fact.

What drives this process of more rapid ageing and earlier disease onset? Probably the insulin primarily but our understanding of all these areas is a bit hazy. We are working to clear the fog. The insulin does this by stimulating our old friend mTOR, there by driving your body down the cellular proliferation and disease pathway.

My comments here refer primarily to those in the majority, the 2/3 of the population who are obese or overweight and who either already have insulin resistance or are at risk of developing it. You are living in a state of carbohydrate poisoning, where your intake exceeds your requirements and the rest just follows on down the train line with the train accelerating until it hits the last stop, where you get off.

If you are thin and exercise a lot or just happen to be

relatively insulin sensitive with low insulin levels then carbohydrate is not an issue for you. Your body uses it rapidly and your insulin levels remain low. There is no real benefit from your going on a low carbohydrate diet that I am aware of.

In summary, restricting carbohydrate with the aim of potentially prolonging life remains unproven in those who are insulin sensitive. The reverse may apply if you look at population studies where longevity is associated with a moderate carbohydrate intake. In those who are insulin resistant a low carb and low to moderate protein diet lowers insulin and glucose levels and should have a very positive flow on effect with disease and life expectancy. In other words, cut down your carbs.

In those of you who are insulin sensitive you may well be able to eat as much carbohydrate as you like, we just don't know. This argument is not "one size fits all"

Protein

Protein intake is critically important in this process of ageing and disease, eclipsing fat and probably even carbohydrate. What is wrong with protein you might stay? We have been told it is an essential part of a healthy diet all our lives. Well indeed it is and it is essential for life. Many of the amino acid building blocks for our body's proteins, such as muscle, are essential in our diet as we cannot make them ourselves. As with many things in life it is all a question of how much is too much. The trouble with living in relatively wealthy countries is we all tend to eat quite a lot of protein. It is the most expensive food source and arguably the tastiest. We even go as far as using protein powders and protein shakes to get really high amounts of protein in the hope it will make our muscles bigger, help us perform in sport and exercise or just keep fit. It is also pushed for weight loss. To some extent it does just that so we see it work and take even more.

A high protein diet is effective in building muscle because it stimulates mTOR. The 3-essential branched chain amino acids; leucine, isoleucine and valine are the most powerful mTOR stimulators known. They will stimulate mTOR even in the absence of high levels of insulin and glucose. When you stimulate mTOR you build muscle and cause cells to grow and divide. The other consequences of this we have discussed repeatedly. As they say, "you cannot have your cake and eat it too."

So how much protein do you actually need to stay healthy? The answer is likely to be a lot less than most of you are now consuming. The guidelines suggest about 0.75 g per kg of body mass. There is no good evidence exceeding 2 g per kg offers any benefit in training or body building but many people take 3g per kg. If I was you I would focus on your lean body mass as fat stores have no use for protein. Your gym trainer can calculate this for you. There seems no sense in working your protein requirement out based on your total body weight, except for those selling you the protein.

If you just want to stay slim and healthy, and body building is not a big deal for you, then I suspect a healthy intake of animal protein, which is high in branched chain amino acids, is no more than about 0.5g per kg lean body weight. This is not the case for those of you who are pregnant or breast feeding where you need at least twice this amount. The other groups to be careful in is the elderly who desperately need muscle bulk to stay mobile and independent, and those of you growing vertically, so be careful restricting their intake below 0.75-1g/kg.

Now I can hear you all saying; "this is rubbish", "my doctor never told me anything like this" and "where is the evidence!" "What can you eat!"

Well hang in there with me for the time being. You understand that people are not mice that you can just put in a cage and test with different diets to see how long they live and what diseases they develop. If we could do this, and I am not suggesting we should, it would give us definite evidence for me to base these claims on.

Where we cannot do studies (with people forced to eat certain diets and followed for years) to prove an idea or hypothesis, we must do detective work and look at the evidence we have available. When we do this in science, medicine or crime scene, we can make mistakes. We can come to the wrong conclusions. There is nothing wrong in keeping an open mind and leaving all the possibilities on the table just in case. I think my conclusions are correct. I will do my best to summarise the evidence available and you can make up your own mind about the guilty party in this discussion. See if you agree or disagree with me.

As we cannot experiment on people let us study flies first and work our way up. Remember the metabolic controller mTOR is very similar no matter if you are talking about flies, mice or people.

We know that dietary restriction prolongs life, presumably by inhibiting mTOR, because in mice genetically bred to have dysfunctional mTOR, dietary restriction has no effect on longevity. Yeasts, fruit flies, worms and mice live longer if you reduce their dietary intake 30-50% below what they would eat if it was up to them. Generally, however the studies also reduce their protein, carbohydrate and fat intake and perhaps it is one of these that is most important rather than calorie restriction.

If you give fruit flies a choice, as perhaps you may expect evolution would dictate, they will eat a diet which maximises their life long egg laying ability. In other words which maximises their reproduction capability and consequently the likelihood of survival of the species. This is a ratio of 1:2 for protein (P): carbohydrate (C).

If you progressively reduce the protein level in their food down to 1:16 for P: C they live progressively longer with the maximal lifespan at 1:16, the lowest level of protein tested. This is even though they eat far more total calories to try and get enough protein from the lower protein food, but despite this, they still lived significantly longer. Those on the highest protein intake ate the lowest total calories and had the shortest lifespan, even though they were slim flies. So perhaps it is not the calorie restriction which is important but the protein restriction.

Lifespan and reproduction in Drosophila: New insights from nutritional geometry PNAS Feb 19, 2008, vol 105 no. 7

Do these effects in flies translate into similar findings in mammals? Well there are mouse models to look at and an excellent study was done in 2014. There were 858 mice in this experiment put into groups on 25 different diets. They were allowed to eat as much as they liked and the variation in the makeup of their food was protein (5-60%), fat (16-75%) and carbohydrate (16-75%). Interestingly the control of their appetite was related mainly to protein and to a lesser extent carbohydrate intake. This resulted in their eating less of the high protein food for example. Fat intake had minimal effect on their appetite which is possibly a bit different to humans. Consequently, the highest calorie or energy intakes were for diets lowest in protein or carbohydrate, with the presumed compensatory over eating targeting a certain amount of protein or carbohydrate.

The results were the same as in the fruit flies. The low protein diet which was high in carbohydrate resulted in a 30% increase in lifespan for the mice. Total intake of calories again had no effect on longevity – it was all about protein. With every increase in protein intake measured (protein concentration in the mouse chow) the lifespan of the mice was shortened.

The researchers note from the literature that "insulin and mTOR are strongly implicated in the relationship between diet and ageing"

Burnett et al 2011

They also note "Branched-chain amino acids (BCAA) are key signals for release of insulin and mTOR activation" Where do you find the highest levels of BCAAs? In animal protein.

Yang et al, 2010

In this study, they looked at mTOR activation in the liver which was maximally influenced by BCAA levels and to a lesser extent glucose. It was maximal (increased 3-fold) on the highest protein diet.

Mitochondrial function (the energy furnace inside

your cells) is gradually impaired with ageing and in this study the mitochondria functioned best on the lowest protein diet. These mice also had the lowest blood pressure, improved insulin sensitivity, higher levels of HDL (good cholesterol), the lowest levels of LDL (bad cholesterol) and lowest levels of triglyceride (blood fat). The mice eating the lowest protein food did not achieve their protein intake target – the protein intake which stopped other mice on higher protein diets eating – despite eating as much as they could manage. This resulted in lower levels of circulating BCAAs in the blood.

As the protein intake increased in the groups of mice the blood BCAAs increased and the liver mTOR activation increased despite low glucose levels. The high protein diets resulted in the lowest food intakes but the highest levels of BCAAs, insulin and mTOR activation with the shortest lifespan.

The diet which was lowest in protein and maximal in carbohydrate (which inhibited appetite in the mice more than low protein high fat combinations) generated the lowest insulin levels (despite high carb intake) and the lowest mTOR activation measured in the liver. It is interesting that high fat low protein mice fared less well than the high carb low protein as fat does not activate mTOR but remember this is not a population of obese type 2 diabetic humans who need to reduce carbs and replace them with fat, they were otherwise fit young laboratory mice. It is also unclear what type of fat they used and this may be important. The results ring the alarm bells about replacing carbs with protein as was common in the Atkins diet of 30 years ago and is still practised today. If you replace protein with fat perhaps you should be careful what type you use, we just don't know.

These results show that in mice, the lowest protein diet was associated with maximal health benefit (despite them eating the most calories!) with minimal mTOR activation and maximal life expectancy. Calorie intake had no effect, so those of you out there doing various fasting techniques such as the 5/2 take note. Those of you taking high protein diets for weight loss and health are also asked to take note.

Cell Metabolism 19, 418-430, March 4, 2014, Solon-Biet et al

So, you may say what has this to do with people? We are not mice! Well remember mTOR is almost identical between mice and people. As discussed, we cannot put people in cages and feed them various diets but we can give them questionnaires and follow them for long periods. Not quite as high a standard of science but it generally shows the same thing. Long term high protein diets, which are often lower in carbohydrate as carbs are replaced by protein, are linked to higher levels of cardiovascular disease and mortality.

One such study looked at 43,396 Swedish women aged 30-49 years at baseline followed for 15.7 years after a dietary questionnaire. They were put into 10 groups dependent on the level of protein intake which correlated inversely with their carbohydrate intake as generally those on a "low carb" diet were replacing carbs with protein. The authors showed that the higher the protein to carbohydrate ratio was, the greater the risk of cardiovascular disease. In cardiovascular disease, they included ischemic heart disease, ischemic stroke, haemorrhagic stroke (bleeding into the brain), subarachnoid haemorrhage (bleeding around the brain), and peripheral vascular disease.

Cardiovascular disease outcomes were 62% more likely in the highest protein compared to lowest protein groups. They conclude high protein low carb diets, although effective for weight loss, may be dangerous to health. What they cannot show is which is important, low carb or high protein. They say it's the carbs. I would argue it is the high protein. In their detailed questionnaires, the "carbs" in the low carb diet group were largely simple sugars and processed foods – which we know are bad. The high carb eaters tended to eat healthy carbs such as vegetables and wholemeal bread with their lower protein diets (and probably were generally more health conscious and exercised more). The higher protein eaters are also likely to have eaten more processed meats.

This study did not report on mortality but as cardiovascular disease is the most common cause of death in western society you can draw your own conclusions.

Low carbohydrate-high protein diet and the incidence of cardiovascular diseases is Swedish women: a prospective cohort study. BMJ 2012 Lagiou et al.

Another population study, or grouping of population studies (meta-analysis) also looked at this. They looked at "low carb" diets and tended to focus again on the "low carb" component but remember these diets typically replace the carbs with protein. We have all been told of the evils of fat all our lives so who would eat that! This meta-analysis of 4 studies involving 272,216 people, showed those on the lowest carbohydrate (likely highest protein) diets were 31% more likely to die from all causes during the study. Interestingly deaths from cardiovascular disease were not statistically significantly more common in this study.

Low-Carbohydrate Diets and All-Cause Mortality; A Systematic Review and Meta-Analysis of Observational Studies PLOS 2013, Noto et al.

It is very difficult to come to any definite conclusions when looking at these population studies because there are literally hundreds of variables at play, any of which may be important (and not discussed). The literature tends to report the "low carb" diets as being potentially bad for you but you must remember, the low carb eaters tended to eat more animal protein and animal fat and less fruit, vegetables and fibre. In the low carb diets, when all pooled together, it may well be the animal protein, red meats and processed meats which convey all the damage and have nothing to do with the "carbs" at all. These are just an inverse marker of animal protein intake. When you do subgroup analysis in the above meta-analysis, the low carb group eating vegetable protein were at lower risk of mortality than average.

A similar meta-analysis when looking at low carb high vegetable intake showed a 20% reduction in all-cause mortality (chance of dying) and a 23% reduction of cardiovascular death compared to the average risk. Again, in the low carb high animal protein intake group the all-cause mortality was 23% higher than average and the risk of cancer related death was 28% higher.

Low-carbohydrate diets and all-cause and cause specific mortality; two cohort studies, Ann Intern Med, Sept 7, 2010, Fung et al

Confusing isn't it! Mice are much easier to work with. I would disagree with the general consensus that low carb diets are bad, based on population studies. I don't think it is about the carbs but rather what you replace them with. If you replace them with high intakes of animal protein, especially processed animal protein and possibly saturated fats, from any source, the outcome is likely to be unfavourable. The trouble is, almost universally this is what people replace their carbs with. When you replace them with low carb vegetables you are actually better off. Vegetables tend to be lower in protein and importantly they are lower in branched chain amino acids (BCAAs).

Remember what the most powerful stimulator of mTOR was?

Lastly let us just look at protein intake and mortality in a group of 6,381 adults over 50 years of age. The group filled out a questionnaire on diet and were divided into 3 groups based on their protein intake, as a % of their calories. The high protein group had greater than 20% of their calories as protein, the moderate group 10-19% and the low protein group less than 10%. They were followed 18 years. Those aged 50-65 years who indicated on questionnaire they were in the high protein group had a 75% increased risk of death from all causes and a 400% increased risk of cancer related death. The increased risk of death was not evident in those over 65 years again suggesting we may need to be cautious restricting protein intake in this elderly group. Over all ages the high protein diet was associated with a 500% increase in diabetes related deaths. The above risk increases were for animal protein only. Protein from plant sources had no effect or an inverse effect in this study.

The high protein diet was associated with high levels of the chemical messenger Insulin like growth factor -1 or IGF-1. This is produced in the liver after stimulation by growth hormone. Those on a low protein diet had lowest levels of IGF-1 in the bloodstream. The investigators show the same thing in the animal model of mice and correlate the findings with the human study. In summary, mice eating high animal protein diets had the highest IGF-1 levels, the highest levels of disease and the shortest lives.

Remember IGF-1 is a powerful stimulator of mTOR. All this starting to sound familiar?

Low Protein Intake Is Associated with a Major reduction in IGF-1, Cancer, and overall Mortality in the 65 and younger but not older population. Cell Metabolism, 2014, Levine et al.

Sorry this is so involved but it is a bit like a crime scene and you need to look carefully at all the evidence, even then you can draw the wrong conclusions. This is why you get so much conflicting advice from the health professionals.

The current guidelines generally do not take into account protein intake, except to ensure you eat enough of it. They are all too busy arguing about fat versus carbohydrate, or the types of fat and the types of carbohydrate. They love terms like "complex carbohydrate" and "good fats" and go on and on and on lecturing you about these. The more they lecture the more confused you get, and the less they have to think. If you say something enough it comes true, doesn't it? "It must be true!" "I've said it a thousand times!"

All this time there is a wolf with big sharp teeth hiding in sheep's clothing right under their noses, unseen by them and waiting to pounce. They tell you not to eat that evil animal fat, don't they? Eat lean meat! What generally comes with that animal fat and may convey all the real negative health consequences in population studies? Could it be animal protein not the fat? Can population studies tell the difference? No. Did your doctor recently say you had early diabetes, high blood pressure, heart disease or cancer? Be careful of a high animal protein diet. Your nutritionist, dietician, or doctor will tell you it is the animal fat you must avoid but I beg to differ. You may be getting older and getting diseases associated with ageing more rapidly than necessary because you are getting the wrong advice.

So, in summary, protein from animal sources with high BCAA levels is a very powerful stimulator of mTOR. The consequences of stimulating mTOR have already been pointed out. A healthy intake of animal protein is probably less than current guidelines recommend and certainly less than most of you in western societies are eating today.

These comments do not apply to certain groups such as growing children and adolescents, pregnant or breast feeding women, the elderly or those recovering from illness or injury. In these situations, you may need extra protein for growth of yourself, your baby or for repair of your body.

The following graph is an attempt to summarise visually the relationship between protein intake and disease throughout your life, for arbitrary protein intakes. The more protein you take in your diet the sooner the diseases are likely to strike. As you get older you get more insulin resistant with all the diseases the metabolic syndrome has to offer coming on tap for you to enjoy. The real question is how rapidly you want this to occur, subjecting yourself to this increasing number of diseases associated with ageing and the metabolic syndrome. I would suggest (and some "experts" would certainly disagree with me) that the higher the protein (particularly animal) intake the more likely these diseases are to occur at a younger age. What diseases you say?

All the diseases listed under the metabolic syndrome of course, they are all intricately related to increasing insulin resistance as you age. These include:

- fatty liver disease

- type 2 diabetes

- Cardiovascular disease (heart attacks and strokes)

- gout

- sleep apnoea

- multiple common cancers...

AGE AND DISEASE FOR DIFFERENT PROTEIN INTAKES

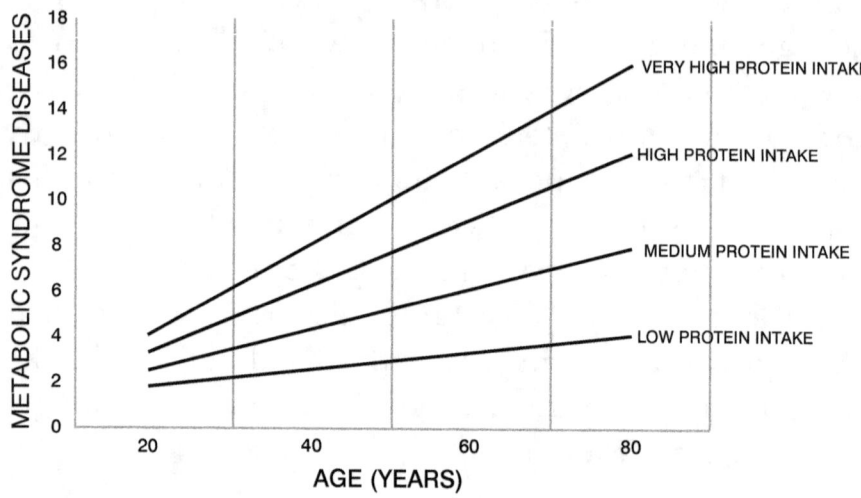

The more diseases you accumulate the more likely you are to die, in other words the younger you are likely to die. The problem is of course the suffering during your life as well which reduces your health span. Your choice. I hope those muscles you can look at in the mirror are worth it.

Fat

Fat has been demonised for generations, particular saturated fat largely from animal sources. Fat and oil are the same thing here and I will use them interchangeably in discussion. For about 70 years we have been saying eat less fat and eat more complex carbohydrate. We even drew pyramids of foods, suggesting which foods to choose, but if you have the metabolic syndrome already, this pyramid is likely to be upside down. This concept is explained in the book "Death by Carbs."

Well that was last century and the obsession was largely with cardiovascular disease. Given that most of us die from cardiovascular disease there presumably were potential implications for life expectancy. That is assuming the hypothesis was correct in the first place. More recent reviews this century suggest the association between dietary saturated fat intake and cardiovascular disease is not as strong as we were led to believe. The levels of saturated fat in the blood stream (where it does matter) does not necessarily correlate very well with the amount of saturated fat in the diet. In many studies, dietary carbohydrate intake correlated a lot better with saturated fat levels in the blood.

For example, a meta-analysis of 21 studies involving 347,747 people followed for between 5-23 years concluded "There is no significant evidence for concluding that dietary saturated fat is associated with an increased risk of coronary heart disease, stroke or cardiovascular disease."

American Journal of Nutrition, Jan 13, 2010, Siri-Tarino et al, USA

There was similar concern about dietary cholesterol and again this has largely been rebuffed as there was never the evidence to support it. The American Heart foundation now say that dietary cholesterol is of no concern with respect to cardiovascular disease risk or serum cholesterol levels. The serum cholesterol is an issue but this topic is complex and has been covered in the previous publication mentioned above. Don't get dietary cholesterol intake and serum cholesterol confused they are different things and do not correlate well at all.

The other issue with fat is it has NIL direct effect on mTOR, at last we have found something that does not affect mTOR!

That being the case it should have no implications for the ageing process? Right?

Unfortunately, few things in life are as simple as we would like them to be. Some fat types probably do have indirect effects on mTOR with potentially life shortening results.

Before we begin this discussion, I would like to subject you to a brief revision about the types of fat so you as understand what I am talking about. Please skip this if you already have a good understanding fat types.

Animal fat or vegetable oil (as they put on food packaging) just doesn't cut it, you need more detail than this basic understanding. You need the simple chemistry. The processed food manufacturing giants would love to keep you in the dark. This maximises their profits!

Fats are make from chains of carbon atoms. The chains

have a CH3 at one end (called the omega end) and a COOH at the other. The simplest is CH3-COOH with no other carbon atoms, this is vinegar or if you like acetic acid. That's right, vinegar is a fat.

Carbon atoms have 4 potential bonding sites you can form bonds with. A bit like a chain of monkeys where they can hold on with either feet or hands to one another, giving them 4 options.

In this chain of carbon there could be 2 bonds between each carbon atom in the chain or just one bond leaving the other potential bond for something on the side of the chain such as a hydrogen molecule.

If all the bonds in the chain of carbon atoms are single, leaving one bond to each side of each carbon atom for hydrogen atoms to attach to the chain, this chain of carbon atoms is said to be saturated with hydrogen. This is what we call saturated fatty acid (SFA) or saturated fat (example; palm oil, coconut oil, butter, animal fat).

If there are multiple double bonds between the carbon atoms, -C=C=C-, the chain is said to be poly (for many) unsaturated fatty acid (PUFA) or polyunsaturated oil. If the first double bond in the chain is in the 3rd position along from the CH3 end it is called omega 3 polyunsaturated oil (example; fish oil, flax seed oil), if it is in the 6th position it is called Omega 6 polyunsaturated oil (example; sunflower oil, rice bran oil).

Most polyunsaturated oils are a combination of omega 3 and omega 6 fatty acids.

If you have only one double bond in the whole chain it is said to be mono (for one) unsaturated fatty acid (MUFA) or monounsaturated oil (example; olive oil, avocado or macadamia nuts.)

So now you know what I am talking about which sort of oil should you eat to maximise your life expectancy? Put simply, we don't know. Having said that, saturated fats are probably not as good for you as those pushing paleo diets or low carb diets would like you to believe. There is also a current craze of "healthy coconut oil" suggesting we should be using more of this and I think "healthy" is the wrong term to use in front of "coconut oil" until we know more.

Starting with the PUFAs these are essential fatty acids, in other words you can't make them yourself and they are essential in your diet for health. They are essential because you make them into numerous other things or chemical messengers in the body, important messengers for fighting infection amongst other things. Some will argue that omega 3 PUFA is better for you than omega 6 because the former is converted into messengers which stop inflammation and the latter into messengers which cause inflammation and this is true but this process is very tightly regulated by the body. In other words, just because you eat a lot of omega 6 fatty acid, the level of the inflammatory messengers in the body will not necessarily rise, as the body will only make as much of these messengers as it needs and no more. A bit like the argument of cholesterol in the diet (where it doesn't matter) not having any significant effect on cholesterol levels in the blood (where it does matter). Both omega 3 and omega 6 PUFA's are probably good for you, but if you want to err on the side of caution use omega 3 fatty acids, the vegetable oil with the most of this and which you can cook with is canola oil. Having said this, a meta-analysis of 20 studies reporting the risk of vascular disease (heart attack and stroke), showed; "Overall, omega-3 PUFA supplementation (fish oil) was not associated with a lower risk of all-cause mortality, cardiac death, sudden death, myocardial infarction or stroke" In other words it didn't matter if you had omega 3 or omega 6 oil.

JAMA 2012; 308(10):1024-1033, Rizos et al.

Mono-unsaturated fatty acid such as olive oil is probably in the same basket as polyunsaturated fatty acids. It is a large part of the Mediterranean diet which seems to confer longevity and health. You can probably have as much of this as you like.

The problems arise when we look at saturated fatty acids such as palm oil or coconut oil and it is not just those Orangutans who are likely to suffer here. Those of you on paleo diets and those on low carb diets tend at times to be a bit like religious fanatics, you may strongly believe something and have no interest in what the science says (in my experience having been shouted down at international meetings discussing this issue.) Many of these dietary "fanatics" say saturated fat is fine and causes no harm, regardless as to whether it is from animal or vegetable sources. They may be right where it is not taken to excess but let me give you some of the science.

We are quite lucky here as we do have data from randomised double blind prospective studies in humans. Not on their effect directly on ageing but on their effect on markers of ageing, diseases such as insulin resistance which are likely to make you die younger.

In a study of 67 people with abdominal obesity, 15% of whom were diabetic the participants were randomised to a diet rich in fatty acid from butter (SFA) or fatty acid from sunflower oil (n-6 PUFA), continuing at a normal overall calorific intake which was the same in both groups. They showed that those on the SFA accumulated more liver fat, developed insulin resistance, had lower levels of good cholesterol (HDL) and higher levels of bad cholesterol (LDL) and higher levels of bad inflammatory markers (TNF and IL1), than those on the PUFA diet. There was no significant change in weight in either group. In other words, this study suggests that if you are obese with diabetes, fatty liver and raised cholesterol, you may benefit from PUFA rather than SFA. Liver fat was reduced and all metabolic parameters improved on PUFA instead of SFA at the same amount. The omega 6 PUFA had no adverse inflammatory effect, and reduced inflammatory markers.

American Journal of Clinical Nutrition 2012, Bjermo et al

Some of you may say this is because the saturated fat came from butter, in other words from an animal source. "Vegetable oil" would have been ok.

Well let's look at palm oil, a saturated vegetable oil (SFA), when compared to sunflower oil (PUFA).

39 well, normal weight individuals were randomised to 7 weeks of 3 muffins per day (an extra 750Kcal), made either with SFA or PUFA. The SFA (palm oil) muffin diet markedly increased the liver fat and abdominal fat levels compared to the PUFA. Both groups were on a high calorie diet but the PUFA actually protected those eating this high calorie diet from increases in liver fat. The liver fat level fell despite the high calorie and high carbohydrate intake. In addition, there was 3 times as much increase in muscle mass in the group on the PUFA diet compared to the SFA diet. They used MRI to measure these levels.

Diabetes, Vol 63, July 2014, Rosqvist et al.

So how quickly and why does this occur with SFA? It is ok to have one biscuit containing palm oil, isn't it?

A German study looked at this with 14 healthy lean

males randomised to receive either a single dose of palm oil about 1 ml per kg body weight or placebo. Those receiving the single dose of palm oil had increases in insulin resistance in the whole body, liver and adipose tissues of up to 34%, a rise in liver fat (triglyceride level) of 35% and a rise in the production of glucose production and output by the liver of 70%. All this following a single dose of palm oil!

In a mouse model, they suggest the palm oil does this by switching on and off genes in the liver. That palm oil seems to be a very powerful poison if one dose can wreak so much havoc on the body's metabolism.

Journal of Clinical Investigation, Jan 2017, Hernandez et al.

Palm oil is the cheapest vegetable oil and in those biscuits and pastries you buy, the "vegetable oil" is very likely to be palm oil, it is the commonest oil used in processed food. It is in almost all processed foods. It is what your fish and chips were fried in when you had takeaway last Friday, it is what the packet chips in supermarket are fried in. If it causes increased liver fat and insulin resistance and is being fed to billions of people worldwide, the potential health consequences and life shortening effect just doesn't bare thinking about. Remember fatty liver is the beginning of the metabolic syndrome, all the rest presumably follows including liver cancer.

What about coconut oil? It is also a vegetable SFA, not identical to palm but similar... You make up your own mind. I don't have any studies to share with you on this but if I were you I would err on the side of caution and avoid it.

These studies are looking at fatty liver disease not longevity but the two issues are related. When you have fatty liver disease with insulin resistance it is the liver that is most resistant to the insulin and is disobeying the instructions from the insulin. Despite insulin messaging the liver to do the reverse, it pumps out glucose (sugar) and triglyceride (fat). This results in higher still insulin levels to try and control the blood sugar and get the liver to behave itself, a bit like yelling at a barking dog when you have asked it to stop barking quietly with no effect! This also results in low levels of good cholesterol (HDL), high levels of blood fats (triglyceride) and subsequently diabetes with higher levels of cardiovascular disease (heart attack and stroke).

High carbohydrate diets are very good at causing fatty liver disease and restricting carbs is a very effective way of treating fatty liver disease. A low carb ketogenic diet results in loss of the fat from the liver and correction of all the metabolic abnormalities. This has been well shown in the literature and is well documented with the evidence quoted in the book "Death by Carbs."

What is now becoming apparent in addition to the story on carbohydrate excess causing fatty liver disease is that saturated fats may be particularly harmful. Diets rich in saturated fats, when compared to unsaturated fats (either MUFA or PUFA), result in fatty liver disease and insulin resistance with all that follows down this pathway including cardiovascular disease and presumably many common cancers. The metabolic syndrome remember is a very good model for accelerated ageing.

If I have made you confused here let me summarise the data for you with respect to diet and make some suggestions about this very important issue.

1. Don't over eat protein, especially from animal sources as it may be sacrificing for your long-term health for short term gains. Remember the exceptions to this include; old and young age, pregnancy, breast feeding, and those recovering from disease or trauma. Generally speaking, I would aim for 0.5 g or less per kg lean body weight, not the recommended 0.75-1g/Kg total body weight.

2. If you already have features of the metabolic syndrome, you are poisoning yourself if you are eating a lot of sugar and other carbs. Read the book "Death by Carbs" This group is probably about 2/3 of the population. If you are thin, fit and insulin sensitive and exercise regularly you do not need to worry about carbs.

3. Choose your fats carefully. You do not need to completely avoid saturated fat by any means but I would not over indulge in this regardless of the source.

Polyunsaturated and monounsaturated fats may be better for you and may delay the onset of the metabolic syndrome and all that it entails. They seem to be able somehow to protect the liver from the carbs causing fatty liver.

So how do I do this and what should I eat to maximise my life expectancy? Well my advice based on my interpretation of the evidence available at this time is;

Lots of Vegetables, lots of unsaturated oils, a small amount of protein, preferably from vegetable sources. No processed foods, they contain palm oil and sugars. If you have features of the metabolic syndrome you should consider restricting grains, starchy vegetables (potato) and sugars as well, and I include here eating large amounts of sweet fruits here. Just like the saturated fat, I don't care where the sugar comes from, your body handles it all the same way. "Vegetable oil" is not all good as I have shown you. There is no such thing as "natural" or "healthy" sugar. Sugar is sugar, processed or not. Wake up and pull your head out of the sand! What planet have you been living on!

An alternative way of thinking about this issue is to change the way you think about upcoming meals. If someone asks what you are having for dinner tonight you are likely to reply, "Steak" and some vegetables on the side, or if you are feeling healthy you reply the fish or the chicken with vegetables. Your whole way of thinking about upcoming meals relates to the protein source in that meal. This influences the way you shop and the way you prepare a meal. The vegetables on the side are an afterthought, whatever you can find left in the fridge will do! You need to turn this around.

You need to think first about the vegetables, stir fried, steamed, curried or whatever and have a small amount of protein on the side. You can use as much polyunsaturated oil as you like to cook those vegetables. The meat, fish or chicken are the garnish on the side. They are not the main component of the meal. Think about what vegetables you are going to shop for and to prepare. They should be the main game here, not the protein source.

Not that complicated, is it?

CHAPTER 8

Exercise

Everyone says you are supposed to exercise to stay healthy but what is the evidence for exercise and does it prolong life? I will discuss this but I think a better way of looking at this is the saying that I've heard before; "exercise adds life to years rather than years to life". The recurring theme in this book is health span not lifespan. The title on the cover of the book was just to trick you into picking the book up to read it.

If you stay fit as you age you are much more likely to have adequate muscle bulk to remain mobile and independent, to look after yourself not have others look after you. Would you really want someone else to have to wipe your backside? Perhaps not a politically correct comment but it is the truth, this is what will happen if you lose your independence. If you remain independent you will be able to get involved in far more activities many of which are social and give you a purpose for living which is arguably more important than the living itself. There is also the added benefit that moderate exercise possibly prevents or delays the onset of that demon of ageing, dementia.

For more than 100, years scientists have been doing research on ageing rates in animal models which is where we usually begin looking at the evidence. Unfortunately for mice and rats they are relatively short lived and cheap to feed and house, making them a good model for humans to use for research. The early studies surprised the investigators back in 1912 as exercise (running in a wheel) appeared to shorten their lives. This resulted in a theory of ageing suggesting that increased rate of energy expenditure shortened lifespan. The assumption was that life span was inversely related to energy expenditure. The current thinking is not along these lines so I apologise to those couch potatoes out there who were getting excited. Rats that exercise regularly do live longer than sedentary rats which tend to become obese, with their food intake outstripping their energy requirements much like their human cousins.

Well as discussed already, you cannot put humans in a cage and make them run in a wheel. You can look at groups who do exercise and groups who do not exercise and match them as far as possible for all other variables.

Meta-analyses of these type of studies demonstrate a clear positive relationship between exercise and life expectancy. Regular physical activity is associated with a reduction overall of about 30% in the risk of all causes of death and the risk of cardiovascular death. It does not matter if you have underlying cardiovascular disease or not, the effect is roughly the same. This risk reduction results in an additional 1-2 years of life when compared to those who engage in little or no physical activity. Data from the Framingham Heart study suggest a benefit of up to 3.7 years of increased lifespan in men and 3.5 years in women who undertook moderate to high physical activity.

New England Journal of Medicine, Paffenbarger et al, 1986

Archives of Internal Medicine, Franco et al, 2005

Meta-analyses of multiple single studies also demonstrate a dose-response relationship. The greater the training volume (which is the exercise intensity x exercise duration) the greater the mortality benefits. In addition to this training volume the greater the intensity of the exercise the greater the benefit in terms of mortality.

For example, looking at endurance athletes competing in Olympic Games longevity is greater by 5.5 years relative to an age matched sedentary group. The same can be shown for cross country skiers or for participants in the Tour de France bicycle race.

Scandinavian Journal of medicine, Grimsmo et al 2011, International Journal of sports medicine, Sanchis-Gomar et al, 2011

More importantly than prolongation of life there are other positive effects of exercise on the ageing process. Cardiorespiratory fitness is a strong predictor of all-cause mortality but clearly if you have good lungs and a good heart you can get up to much more mischief and potential enjoyment in those years you have left.

Sarcopenia refers to age related loss of muscle, in terms of volume, strength and speed of contraction. Exercise has been shown to prevent or delay this loss again leading to greater independence. It's a bit hard to enjoy life to the fullest if you cannot get out of bed or up from the couch because your muscles are too weak to lift you. Strength or weight training is the best way to prevent this muscle loss and one would also potentially remove restriction in protein intake if sarcopenia was becoming an issue.

Osteoporosis refers to thinning of your bones which occurs with ageing in all of us. Exercising particularly heavy resistance training with weights, or exercises which involve weight bearing or your whole-body weight are the best way to combat the osteoporosis and strengthen bones. Exercise has not been shown to reduce fracture risk however which is a point of concern. I would suggest this is not surprising however as it is a bit difficult to break your hip if you are sitting on a couch watching mountain climbing on TV compared to someone who goes mountain climbing! Clearly there are other factors as well which come into play including adequate intake of calcium and vitamin

D in the elderly, but I would rather be the one out doing the mountain climbing!

Matuitas 73(2012), Gremeaux et al

In addition, regular physical activity has unequivocally been shown to reduce the risks of cardiovascular disease, stroke, hypertension, type 2 diabetes, obesity, bowel cancer, breast cancer, anxiety and depression. It also reduces the risk of falls and the likelihood of injury associated with falls.

Circulation, 2007, Nelson et al.

For about 40 years there has been increasing evidence in the literature that regular exercise may improve your brain function and prevent or delay the onset of dementia with ageing. A study in 1984 showed that in people aged 55-70, 4 months of aerobic exercise training improved multiple neuropsychological testing scores compared with sedentary controls.

Neurobiology of ageing, Dustman et al.

Another study showed that in 60-79 year old's, 6 months of aerobic fitness training can increase brain volume particularly in regions associated with age-related decline compared to controls. Significant increases in brain volume in both grey and white matter were found in those who participated in aerobic fitness training but not in those who participated in a stretching and toning (nonaerobic) control group.

The brain volume was assessed with MRI scanning and the study did not look at brain function issues.

J Gerontology, 2006, Colcombe et al.

Looking at brain function, another study of 1740 people aged over 65 without evidence of dementia were followed up for 6.2 years. The incidence of dementia was 13 per 1000 person-years in the group who exercised more than 3 times per week and 20 per 1000 person years in the group that exercised less than 3 times per week. The lower the performance level of the participants or if you like the more difficult it was for them to exercise the greater the benefit of the exercise. In this study, the reduction in the dementia risk was 40% and was highly statistically significant (p=0.004). They only measured frequency of activity, not intensity or amount of exercise. Now you can criticise any one study but when they all start to say the same thing they are likely to be reflecting real effects.

Annals of Internal Medicine, 2006, Larson et al.

A theoretical reason exercise may be causing life prolongation goes again back to mTOR and the fact that exercise reduces insulin resistance, glucose and insulin levels, reducing stimulation of the enzyme complex. This is academic. The fact is exercise really does adds years to life and life to years, but I would be focused more on the latter.

Exercise needs to be part of the equation of disease prevention and life prolongation which are really one and the same thing. It seems the more intense the exercise is, within the limits of not injuring yourself, the better.

CHAPTER 9

Medications and Supplements which may delay the ageing process

Rapamycin

This is the drug with which discussion on ageing began and from which mTOR takes its name. I have touched on it in the discussion in the chapter on mTOR. Rapamycin has been shown to prolong life in all animal models tested including mice (mammals) with obvious implications for humans. There is argument as to the mechanism for this with some scientists believing it prevents or delays cancer related deaths rather than slowing ageing. This resulting in a longer life span as in many mouse models the primary cause of death is cancer. In humans, it is only used as an immunosuppressant in organ transplantation and in coronary artery stents to stop blockage caused by the artery lining called endothelium growing into the stent.

Interesting areas for further investigation are inhibition of cancer, with the potential for newer more specific drugs to treat cancer, and the effect on cognitive decline with ageing in mice. This is a good model for dementia and it appears that rapamycin like drugs prevent neurological decline in learning and memory as well as motor function. In mice, it has also been shown to reverse early established cognitive deficits, restoring them to normal function. It had no effect in late stage disease. Perhaps it may help in early in Alzheimer's disease in humans?

Treatment in mice also appeared to reduce the protein plaques and tangles in the mouse brains which are associated with the onset of dementia and to activate autophagy suggesting this may be the mechanism by which it works in preventing animal models of dementia. It also improves blood flow in the brain.

There is limited data in humans but one study looking at heart transplant patients treated with a Rapamycin derivative, Everolimus, showed after 4 weeks on the new treatment (switching to this from another drug), there were significant improvements in memory, depression and executive function on testing of these with standardised tests.

So why are we not using this class of drug more widely? Well because of their side effects. These drugs cause mouth ulcers, skin rashes, immunosuppression predisposing to infection, high blood sugar (diabetes) and high blood fats. This appears in part because when used long term they indirectly inhibit mTOR-2 rather than just mTOR-1. The mTOR-2 complex is important in insulin sensitivity and inhibiting it causes diabetes. If you need them because you have had a heart transplant then this may be a small price to pay but if you are currently well it is too much. There is a rush on to produce new drugs without these side effects and the first drug company to do so will make a lot of money.

Metformin

Metformin like drugs or biguanides have been around since the time of the ancient Egyptians when the herb Goat's rue or French lilac was used to make tea to treat frequent urination, a symptom of diabetes. The chemical Metformin was derived from this herb in the 1920s and found to be useful for diabetes in the 1950s. Since then it has become the first line treatment for type 2 diabetes for good reason.

Metformin has been recognised in multiple studies to result in healthier and longer lifespans in mice and other animal models, leading to consideration of its use to prolong health span in humans. No studies have yet been done in humans who are not diabetic and all our data comes from looking at its use in humans with diabetes. This time I will keep the discussion to human studies considering a few different issues;

cardiovascular disease the most common cause of death in our society, cancer, the demon dementia and overall life expectancy. The focus as always is quality of life lived, rather than length of life however you are likely to get the latter free at no extra charge as well.

Cardiovascular disease is the leading cause of death in Western society. If you have type 2 diabetes this risk increases a massive 200-400 percent above the rest of the population. This results in 75% of type 2 diabetics dying from a cardiovascular event. It is not entirely clear why the risk is increased so much however insulin resistance is likely to play a pivotal role, suggesting the entire metabolic syndrome is linked into this risk increase as well. Insulin resistance, type 2 diabetes and cardiovascular disease are strongly linked to ageing. If you can slow the ageing rate one would expect you to delay the onset of these diseases.

Am J Cardiol. 1999, Haffner et al.

Multiple subsequent studies have shown a reduction in cardiovascular disease in diabetics who take Metformin. An English study randomising diabetics to Metformin or diet alone showed a reduction in the risk of having a heart attack of 39% in the Metformin group at a median follow up of 11 years and 33% at 20 years. This study showed a reduced all-cause mortality of 36% in those on Metformin. The effect did not appear related to diabetic control as the blood sugars in the 2 groups were comparable.

UKPDS Lancet, 1998

In another study of greater than 20,000 people with diabetes and known atherosclerosis (cardiovascular disease) Metformin use was associated with a 24% lower chance of dying from all causes

REACH, Arch Intern Med, 2010.

An added advantage of Metformin use is that it is consistently associated with weight loss of 2-3 kg within 4-6 months of starting, presumably because it seems to reduce appetite and food intake. There is concern that because it is excreted by the kidneys that it is not safe to take in kidney failure patients but there is argument about this issue as they also potentially have a lot to gain as many diabetics have kidney failure with the diabetes. The same is true of heart failure where Metformin has been shown to reduce the risk of death in animal models of diabetic mice and in humans. In the REACH study above Metformin lowered the risk of dying from heart failure by 31% compared to those not taking it. At least 5 large studies have shown an improved outcome in patients with heart failure taking Metformin.

Diabetes, 2011, Xie et al.

A recent meta-analysis of 204 studies involving more than 1.4 million people showed that Metformin use was associated with a 30-40% reduction in the risk of dying of heart disease in diabetics when compared to other medications used to treat the diabetes.

Annals of Internal Medicine, April 2016, Maruthur et al.

There are other studies I could mention but they all show much the same thing with a reduction in the risk of dying from cardiovascular disease and a reduction in all-cause mortality of around 30-35%, over periods as short as 5-6 years, when used in diabetic patients. The most dramatic finding was in a UK study where the obese type 2 diabetics with multiple co-morbidities (other diseases), who were over 70 and on Metformin outlived the "healthy" non-diabetic less obese controls not taking the Metformin.

Bannister et al, 2014, Diabetes. Obes. Metab.

Too many figures I'm sorry but you get the message. If you are a type 2 diabetic and you are not taking Metformin you need to ask your doctor why.

What about Metformin treatment and cancer? At least in theory, as Metformin inhibits mTOR and consequently cell growth, and as mTOR is over produced by cancer cells, you may expect it to be beneficial in treating and preventing cancer. Indirectly it also reduces the levels of insulin and IGF-1 both important growth factors for cancer. They are both a bit like fertiliser for the weeds.

Human studies in diabetics taking Metformin report a 31% reduction in cancer incidence (new cancers) and a 34% reduction in the chance of dying from cancer,

Gandini et al, 2014.

Numerous observational studies have shown a reduction in cancer incidence and cancer related mortality in diabetics taking Metformin with the strength of the effect related to the time of exposure to Metformin. This applies to almost every common cancer you care to name but additionally those taking Metformin seem to respond better to cancer treatment with higher responses to treatment shown for breast cancer and oesophageal cancer in those taking this treatment. There have been some negative studies (no effect) related to prostate and pancreatic cancer but most studies show a positive effect. It does not seem to matter if you are talking about animal models, cancer cells growing in a dish in the laboratory or human studies, Metformin seems to inhibit cancer growth.

Metformin is a small molecule and can cross the blood brain barrier and get into the brain. When one looks at dementia and Metformin you find similar positive results. Again, diabetics are the groups studied as they are the ones on the Metformin, they also have about a 50% increased rate of dementia when compared to the non-diabetic population.

A study conducted in Singapore showed a 51% reduction in cognitive decline (as assessed by mini-mental studies) in those taking Metformin compared to those not and the effect was more pronounced the longer the drug was taken, after 6 years the reduced risk was 70%.

Ng et al. 2014

Other large observational studies have shown similar effects with lower rates of dementia in diabetics treated with Metformin when compared to other medication. When compared to the standard therapy of sulfonylureas there was a 22% reduction on Metformin and when compared to another drug type, a thiazolidinedione the reduction was greater than 400% in dementia risk.

Chang et al, 2014

In a study of diabetics over 55 years comparing Metformin and Insulin over 5 years the Metformin resulted in a 20% reduction in dementia and insulin resulted in a 28% increase in risk for dementia. Not surprising really when you look at the effects of Metformin and insulin on mTOR.

In a study looking at dementia and Parkinson's disease development in just over 6000 diabetic Veterans followed for 5.3 years there was a progressive reduction in the risk of either dementia or Parkinson's disease with increasing time of treatment with Metformin, from a risk of 2.47 per 100 person years in the first year to a tiny 0.49 per 100 person years if treated for over 4 years. Overall those on Metformin had a 30-40% reduction in the risk of dementia or Parkinson's disease

Qian Shi, June 2016, Clinician Reviews

This has led to studies using Metformin to treat dementia. In a group of 80 non-diabetic patients with mild dementia Metformin led to significant cognitive improvement in some areas after 12 months. This is preliminary unpublished data.

Luchsinger et al. 2016.

This has also been shown in mice where spatial learning tests in mazes shows mice treated with Metformin have significantly improved memory for finding hidden rewards. There is also data from the lab suggesting Metformin can stimulate growth in human neural stem cells, in other words the growth of nerve cells. Perhaps this offers hope in other forms of brain injury recovery? Further studies will tell.

At this time, it looks very likely that Metformin may help to protect your brain from the effects of ageing, at least if you are a diabetic. More studies in non-diabetics are in the pipe line. The effect does not correlate with lowering blood sugar so may be applicable to non-diabetics as well.

There appear to be many ways Metformin potentially prolongs your health span, reducing your risk cardiovascular disease, cancer and dementia, at least in diabetics. Does it prolong your lifespan as well?

It certainly does if you are a worm, a fruit fly or a mouse. In these models, it leads to a longer healthier life, increasing health span and lifespan. In different strains of mice this increase is small at about 6% but was statistically significant, correlating to about 4 years in humans. We do not have data in human studies to prove this as yet but it looks promising.

Remember Metformin decreases levels of insulin and IGF-1 which reduces mTOR activation. It also directly inhibits mTOR and it indirectly inhibits mTOR by increasing AMP kinase levels. If you can inhibit mTOR it is likely you will live longer but this remains to be proven in human studies. Metformin does indeed inhibit mTOR in multiple ways.

The last question which of course we must ask here is: "Is Metformin safe to take long term?"

Well there is some debate about this but I think the answer is yes, yes and yes. It has been used for over 60 years with an excellent safety record. Monitoring of side effects in clinical trials is very close. In 2012 18,000 patient years of follow up had been accrued and 20% of this cohort was 70 years or older. There were no cases of lactic acidosis reported and no cases of significant hypoglycaemia.

Diabetes Prevention Program Research Group 2012.

Lactic acidosis refers to a high concentration of lactic acid in the blood, usually because of some catastrophic life threatening event such as severe trauma or sepsis (infection) but may also occur with the group of medications to which Metformin belongs. This scares doctors because patients have quite a high risk of dying from the acidosis or more likely from the cause of the acidosis. Metformin is excreted by the kidneys and in renal failure the levels in the blood may become very high increasing theoretically increasing the risk of this serious disease. Lactic acidosis also occurs in Metformin overdose.

As I see it, there are a few problems with the current guidelines here. They essentially say if you have significant kidney disease you cannot have Metformin.

When little doctors are growing up into big doctors they are taught the first rule of medicine is "do no harm!" and the second rule is probably "follow guidelines don't question them!". Unfortunately harm is unavoidable when one is trying to balance risks in medicine or in life generally.

The problem is if something happens because of the doctor's action, for example starting a patient on a drug, the doctor feels very bad, is worried he may end up in court and says, "I'll never do that again!"

What about something happening because of the doctor's inaction?! Much easier for the doctor to say, "well I didn't do it!" We know from the UKPDS study above that over 10 years, those diabetics taking Metformin had a 39% reduced risk of a heart attack and a 36% reduced risk of dying! In other words, 1/3 of all the deaths, which occurred in the group not on

Metformin were potentially avoidable, if all patients were taking Metformin.

Meta-analyses of 347 trials of diabetics on Metformin, more than half of which included patients with kidney disease, with >70,000 years of patients on Metformin showed NOT ONE CASE of lactic acidosis.

Salpeter et al, Cochrane database 2010

Metformin use in diabetics is said to be associated with a risk of lactic acidosis about 3-4 per 100,000 patient years which is effectively the same as the incidence in the general population. Which would you rather; an increased risk 1/3 of death over 10 years off Metformin vs a risk of 0/70,000 on Metformin of getting lactic acidosis which carries about a 25% mortality if it does occur?

Am I missing something here?? A choice between actual increased risk of dying of 1/3 if you follow guidelines and don't take metformin vs 1/280,000 if you do not follow guidelines and take metformin with kidney disease. Rough figures as not all the patients above had kidney disease.

I am not saying if you are diabetic with kidney disease you must take Metformin, I am just saying you should discuss the relative risks with your doctor. Personally, I feel you should be on it at a lower dose and be carefully monitored. If you have severe kidney disease however we don't know the answer and I would avoid it until we do. My comments refer to mild to moderate kidney disease only. Generally, it is very safe.

Should we all be taking it once we are over 50 years of age? We don't know because we do not have the high-quality trials to prove benefit in normal people yet. Only diabetics. The medical profession will not recommend something until we have this firm data (another generally sensible rule taught to little doctors). We have broken this rule in the past and got the answer wrong. Vitamin A an antioxidant vitamin seemed like a good idea in smokers to reduce the risk of lung cancer – at least on theoretical grounds. That was until we realised when it was put to the test in a big trial in smokers, it actually increased the risk of lung cancer. The trial had to be stopped. The trouble with waiting for the high-quality evidence on Metformin is it may well come too late for you as an individual. The protective effect does not seem to relate to blood sugar level, it is something else other than diabetic control.

Do I take Metformin? Yes. I take it at a low dose primarily because of concern about the demon dementia. No, I'm not diabetic or insulin resistant.

Should you take it? I suggest you discuss this with your doctor, read some of the references I have given you and watch for more studies, then you decide when you feel fully informed – if your doctor agrees. The internet is a very powerful tool but use something like google scholar and stick to the medical journals. I have tried to give you the evidence on which I base my opinions in this discussion but remember we are all fallible. We are still waiting for the studies of benefit in normal non-diabetic people but they are not likely to be far away.

Aspirin

Aspirin is another old drug. Similar compounds referred as salicylates have been extracted from plants such as willow leaves for more than 2000 years. Willow bark extract was used for joint pains and fevers since the mid 1700's. In 1853 chemists synthesised acetylsalicylic acid or aspirin for the first time and in 1897 scientists at the drug firm Bayer had begun large scale production.

Aspirin, like many drugs, has numerous effects on different parts of the body. It is useful in the treatment of fever, pain and inflammation. If given as soon as possible after a heart attack it decreases the risk of sudden death. It can also be used long term to lower the risk of heart attacks, strokes and blood clots. It reduces the risk of some common cancers.

Like Metformin, Aspirin inhibits mTOR and is an activator of AMP kinase, which indirectly inhibits mTOR further and controls intracellular energy homeostasis and metabolism. It inhibits inflammation by inhibiting production of some prostaglandins and this makes your blood less sticky and less likely to clot. These things make it a very promising drug when considering preventing ageing and thereby preventing common age related disease.

Aspirin reduces the incidence of cardiovascular events by 12% in both the general population and high risk groups.

Lancet 2009 Balgent et al.

When you look at cancer, there is a lot of evidence in the literature which suggests regular aspirin use prevents new cancers developing (reduces cancer incidence) and reduces the risk of dying from cancer. As one would expect this effect takes about 3-5 years to become apparent. The reported risk reductions in case control studies, in incidence and mortality, are strongest and most established in bowel cancer at 25-63% but also seen in oesophageal cancer 22-73%, stomach cancer 23-62%, pancreatic cancer 0-20%, lung cancer 0-27%, prostate cancer 9-14%, breast cancer 2-20% and uterine cancer. Where I have included zero in the risk reduction I mean that some studies showed no effect. Given many of these are common cancers the overall cancer risk reduction by taking regular aspirin is estimated at about 25%. It is suggested the benefit-harm profile favours the use of aspirin.

Annals of Oncology 2015, Cuzick et al.

The evidence for low dose aspirin preventing dementia

is not there. There have been negative studies looking at this, such as the Women's health study in >6000 women followed for 10 years with a dose of 100mg alternate days having no effect.

BMJ 2007.

This result obviously does not exclude higher doses being effective but we do not have that data and it cannot be recommended for this indication. Vascular dementia, presumed related to disease in the arteries in the brain is a situation where one would expect it to work but again there is no good evidence that it is effective. It is effective however in stroke and heart attack, and presumably vascular dementia may not relate to "multiple small strokes" as doctors have assumed to be the cause.

Does aspirin prevent ageing in humans? We don't know. There is no argument it reduces some forms of cardiovascular disease and cancer. It has been shown to prolong life in male mice and worms but not as yet in human beings.

What are the potential problems with taking aspirin? Predominantly inflammation and ulcer formation in the gut, which can have fatal outcomes related to bleeding or perforation of the gut. There is a condition in children and adolescents, Reyes syndrome, involving acute liver and brain disease which has been reported more commonly following aspirin. This can be fatal and is a warning against using this drug in childhood.

Should you be taking it? Only at low dose (75-100mg daily) and there is still a risk of harm from gut ulcers or bleeding but this is probably outweighed by the reduction in cardiovascular and cancer events. Again discuss this with your doctor. If you are taking higher doses you should probably be on other drugs as well to protect your stomach from the potential negative effects of the aspirin.

Caffeine

Caffeine has been shown to prolong the lifespan and health span in yeasts and in worms in a similar fashion to rapamycin. It has been shown to be a selective inhibitor or mTOR-1 without inhibiting mTOR-2 in the yeast model.

Molecular Microbiology July 2008.

In mice and rat models of Parkinson's disease and Alzheimer's disease it prevents these and improves memory. It has even been shown to reverse dementia in mice.

Now before you fall asleep with all these figures and references, take note, this has significant implications for human beings.

Caffeine is the most widely consumed psychoactive drug in the world today. Chronic moderate consumption has been linked with reduced risk for developing neurodegenerative age associated diseases including dementia overall, Alzheimer's type dementia and Parkinson's disease. Its consumption has been associated with reduced incidence of fatty liver disease, type 2 diabetes, inflammatory disease, stroke and reduced overall mortality in elderly population studies.

The trouble with humans again is the difficulty in looking at caffeine consumption in isolation. One study looked at coffee consumption as a marker. The trouble with this is coffee drinkers are more likely to smoke so this risk must be adjusted for. In review of a study involving more than 400,000 people and 52,000 deaths coffee consumption was associated with reduction in total and cause specific mortality.

Total mortality (the chance of dying) fell progressively as coffee consumption increased, and was reduced by 15% at 4-5 cups daily. This finding was highly statistically significant. Looking at disease specific deaths there was a reduction in death from heart disease, lung disease, stroke, diabetes, injuries and accidents. There did not appear to be any significant reduction in the risk of cancer related death. They make the point that coffee contains at least 1000 compounds other than caffeine, in other words this does not prove it is the caffeine but animal models we have would suggest it may be. We know caffeine inhibits mTOR.

Association of Coffee Drinking with Total and Cause-Specific Mortality, New England Journal of Medicine, Freedman et al, 2012

Natural products – Fruit and Vegetables

You may have noted that all the substances described above are natural in that they come originally from nature in one way or another. The beneficial effect of many natural fruits and vegetables on health span and life span may well relate to their effect on the mTOR pathways, and this in part explain their beneficial effect on your health. I am not suggesting we know all the biochemical pathways by which they exert their effects, but what we do know suggests they may well be helpful in inhibiting ageing and all that goes with it including diabetes, cardiovascular disease and cancer. Those that I list here have predominantly been shown to have anti-cancer effects and are felt to work through the mTOR and associated pathways. They include

Flavonoids - oranges, apples, cherries, grapes, strawberries, onions, parsley, broccoli, green pepper tomatoes, tea and wine.

Curcumin - The pigment in the spice Turmeric. This has numerous anticancer effects in testing, the mechanism for many of these are not understood yet.

Indoles - Broccoli, cauliflower, cabbage and Brussel sprouts

Isoflavones - Soybeans

Quercetin - Tea, onions, red grapes and apples

Resveratrol - Red grapes and red wine

Anthocyanins - Phenolic pigments in bright blue or red berries, cherries grapes and purple vegetables

This list is not complete, I am just giving some examples which have been well tested.

In cancer models in animals, or in the laboratory, these compounds variably inhibit the development of cancer in many cell lines, growth of the cancer, spread or metastasis of the cancer and the ingrowth of blood vessels into the cancer necessary for bringing the cancer oxygen and nutrition.

So, your mother was right. You should eat your vegetables!

CHAPTER 10

The Sun

C learly the sun is the only reason we are having this discussion or if you like that you are reading the book. I prefer to think of it as a discussion between the two of us and that is how I like to write. The sun is the reason life exists on this planet. Could it be that it may have something to do with the length of your life as well as allowing you to live?

I have thought about this issue for many years. After nearly 30 years of medical practice working in Northern Australia I have seen a lot of sun and a lot of sun related skin damage. When I first moved up from Melbourne in the south to Townsville in the north I could not believe the level of sun damage to the skin of some individuals. I was literally speechless. Since then this dramatic level of solar skin damage has become relatively "normal" to me and doesn't get a second glance.

In my line of medicine, I have seen a lot of old people, as doctors we tend to see more older people as they are the ones with disease as discussed earlier in the book. Age and many western diseases as I keep suggesting to you are one and the same thing.

One thing has struck me over and over and over again. Every time I see someone over 90 years of age who is very well, thin, mobile and quick witted they seem to come from cattle stations "out west" and have a history of working in the open all their lives. Their brains and everything else on the inside of them is often in very good shape but their skin looks horrific due to the degree of sun damage. They have often had more than 100 small skin cancers burnt off or cut out but they remain well active and often still work in the cattle yards! My assumption has always been that they are so well because of their sun exposure and raised vitamin D levels but I have never found evidence in the literature to prove this. Perhaps there is another reason which I am missing and my assumptions are incorrect.

Writing this book has made me get off my backside and look into the issue. It seems odd that studies about the sun seem to come from places without any and I will quote a few of these studies. Perhaps it is because if there is very little sun the potential diseases arising from lack of exposure will be more obvious.

We have all been taught we must be very scared of the

Sun and this is for a good reason, cancer. In Australia, our public health message is; Slip, Slop, Slap. Meaning slip on a shirt, slop on some sunscreen and slap on a hat. I have no argument with this and if followed, particularly by children and adolescents, it is likely to save lives. Nothing is ever as simple as it appears at first glance however.

When one looks at skin cancer related to UV light exposure, we group the cancers into two types. Non-melanoma skin cancer (basal cell carcinoma and squamous cell carcinoma) and melanoma skin cancer. The grouping is important because melanoma kills people much more commonly than non-melanoma skin cancer. The risk factors for these is probably a bit different as well. Non-melanoma skin cancer is associated with the total exposure to UV light in your lifetime where melanoma is more associated with the number of episodes of severe sunburn, particularly in childhood and adolescence. There is more sun in Northern Queensland than Southern Queensland but the melanoma rate is higher in the south, even though as many people work outdoors in the North. This is probably because it is too hot to lie on the beach where I live and if you do you risk being eaten by a saltwater crocodile. In the South, it is cooler and the beaches are beautiful, there are no crocodiles, and people lie in the sun until they look like a cooked lobster. Frequent use of tanning beds achieves the same thing with respect to your risk for melanoma and cooked crustacean appearance.

So, let's look at non-melanoma skin cancer. A Danish study looked at over 70,000 patients having a basal cell carcinoma (BCC) removed and followed them over 10 years comparing them to a matched population of just under 400,000 controls without BCC. If you had a BCC removed, the least risky and commonest type of skin cancer, you are 10% less likely to die over the next 10 years than your mate who has not had one removed. Presumably this BCC removal reflects your greater sun exposure as does the reduced mortality.

Acta Derm Venereol, 2010, Jensen et al.

A Swedish study looked at UV exposure, by questionnaire, and mortality among women. Over 15 years they followed 38,472 women aged 30-49 when enrolled. During which time 754 of them died.

They looked at the all-cause mortality or chance of dying, with women who got sunburnt twice or more per year during adolescence, compared to those sunburnt once or less. Those sunburnt twice or more were 30% less likely to have died. Women who spent more than one week per year on sunbathing vacations, between the ages of 10 and 39 years were also 30% less likely to have died from all causes or from cardiovascular disease. There was no effect on cancer related mortality. Solarium use was associated with an increase in all-cause mortality of 90%.

Note solarium use also increases vitamin D so perhaps the sun does something else and it's not all about vitamin D?

These findings were highly statistically significant, in other words likely to be correct.

American Association for Cancer Research, 2011, Yang et al.

Another Swedish study more recently has shown similar findings. They followed 29,518 women for 20 years primarily looking at melanoma. They were given a questionnaire at the start of the study.

When they compared those reporting the lowest versus the highest sun exposure, the life expectancy in the lowest sun exposure group was reduced by up to 1.3 years in non-smokers and 2.1 years in smokers, by the age of 60 years. In the older groups the effect was much greater, roughly halving the mortality from all causes and from cardiovascular disease in both smokers and non-smokers who had the most sun exposure compared to the least.

The startling finding was when one looked at the graphed results, comparing non-smoking sun avoiders with smoking sunbathers the mortality was the same! In other words, not going out in the sun puts you at the same risk of death as smoking! Not really fair, is it?

This study showed a dose dependent reduction in the risk of dying from all causes and from cardiovascular disease with increasing sun exposure. The group with the highest life expectancy and the lowest risk of death in this study were the ones who got the non-melanoma skin cancers. Their risk was reduced 4-fold or 400%. They were also the ones with the greatest sun exposure. Looking at melanoma you were more likely to die if you had this but the risk of dying if you got a melanoma was 4 times higher in those who avoided the sun compared to those who had the most exposure. Melanoma was much more common in those sun exposed individuals however by a factor of 10 times.

Those most sun exposed who got melanoma were no more likely to die overall than controls without skin cancer of any sort. In other words, if you get a melanoma associated with sun exposure it seems to have a more benign course in this study, but they did get far more melanomas with increased sun exposure. Putting that another way; there were 4 out of the 14 patients with melanoma in the sun avoidance group who died compared with 14 out of 126 patients with melanoma in the highest sun exposure group who died.

Journal of Internal Medicine, Oct 2016, Lindqvist et al.

Interestingly since the 1980s we have had data suggesting sun exposure may be protective for disease. Many studies have shown a seasonal difference in the risk for heart attacks, strokes and for venous blood clots (pulmonary emboli) comparing summer and winter.

The risk is lowest in the summer when the sun is shining. In the tropics, the risk is the same all year round.

We know that UV radiation is related to altitude and increases by about 10% for every 300m increase in altitude. If the sun protects you from cardiovascular disease, one would expect those people living at higher altitude to have lower risks of cardiovascular disease and possibly cancer. When you look at these populations this is indeed the case. Once you go over about 300m mortality rates begin to decline. The effect seems mainly to be on heart disease, which is our biggest killer. In the 1960s doctors performing autopsies on people who had died in the Andes Mountains reported a zero incidence of disease of the coronary arteries, they did not find one person who had died of a heart attack.

In New Mexico, it was noted males were 72% less likely to die from heart disease than those living at sea level and the same was found in the mountains of Greece, and the Alps of Switzerland, France, Italy and Austria. The risk of dying from cardiovascular disease was reduced by 60-70% in some of the communities and the risk of some cancers also seemed lower. Clearly there are factors other than UV radiation at play here, with more exercise and altered diet but I wouldn't mind betting the Sun is the primary issue. Manual workers on farms at sea level often work hard but don't have this great a reduced mortality. The effect seemed more pronounced in males, possibly because they spend more time outdoors. Multiple studies say the same thing, living at higher altitude seems to protect you from cardiovascular disease, stroke and some cancers.

The other thing that changes UV radiation rates is latitude. In Europe when you move south from Finland in the north to Italy or Greece in the south, there is a progressive drop in the rates of cardiovascular disease. There is a huge amount of discussion as to why this should be the case and most of this discussion centres on diet. The Finnish diet being largely saturated fat and no vegetables and the Mediterranean diet being all olive oil, fruit and vegetables. I suspect diet is part of the equation explaining this but what seems to be overlooked every time in all the discussion? The Sun. There is an inverse relationship between solar radiation and mortality as you move north or south. They are both relatively straight lines on a graph. The higher the solar radiation levels in the European continent, the lower the incidence of cardiovascular disease mortality. I am sticking to Europe as this continent is largely "Westernised" so they have similar but certainly not identical, lifestyles, health care opportunities and access to fast food.

So perhaps the factor in the Mediterranean diet which protects you from heart disease is not "diet" at all? Just food for thought.

You might expect airline pilots who spend a lot of time at high altitudes to have a lower mortality than the rest of the population, despite their very sedentary work and the other forms of "harmful" radiation at this altitude. This is the case in some studies. A group of American airline pilots aged 60 at retirement were followed and found to live 5 years longer than matched controls they were compared with. Not all studies agree on this however.

Federal Aviation Administration, US Department of Transportation 1995.

There are multiple other benefits of sun exposure which don't even get considered while we are all running for cover because of the issues related to skin cancer. These include an antidepressant effect with elevation of mood, possibly related to regulation of the biological clock improving sleep and mood. There are also effects regulating the immune system with a reduction in flu and other infectious illnesses during summer months and documented improved mood during summer. The immune regulation may also be the reason that the incidence of autoimmune diseases such as SLE or Lupus falls progressively as one moves towards the equator from the north or the south. Seasonal affective disorder is a real entity. It means if you move away from the equator people are more likely to get depressed in winter.

Getting adequate sleep is very important and if sun exposure helps this by setting the circadian rhythm or biological clock it has implications for cortisol secretion, an adrenal hormone, and other metabolic messengers which causes insulin resistance. In other words, shift work, where your internal clock is misaligned and repetitively changed messes up your metabolism and has been shown to put normal people into the pre-diabetic state with marked insulin resistance and subsequently higher insulin levels. This may be why there is an increased risk of obesity, diabetes and cardiovascular disease in shift workers. This may go hand in hand with more rapid ageing.

PNAS 2009 Scheer et al.

Are some of the effects of sunlight mediated by vitamin D?

We don't know for sure but the general consensus is that they may be related to vitamin D production in the skin. There is not much vitamin D in your diet and it is estimated that 90% of your requirements come from production in the skin from an interaction between UVB radiation and a cholesterol like compound. This produces what we call vitamin D3 which is then activated in the liver and the kidney to its fully active from.

Receptors for vitamin D are present in almost all the

tissues in the body, not just bone. It is necessary for absorption of calcium and phosphate from the gut for strong and healthy bones but has numerous other effects. Low levels of vitamin D in the blood are associated with higher risks of cardiovascular disease, cancer, infections and autoimmune disease in many studies. Low levels of vitamin D are associated with a significantly higher total mortality (chance of dying) of about 31% in a review of 11 different studies.

We set the "normal" lower limit at about 50 nmol/l but mortality continues to fall up to levels of about 90nmol/l. Increases after this level do not seem to convey any benefit and may even be toxic, with higher mortality at higher vitamin D levels. In other words, it is a U-shaped graph.

How does it work? Well as usual we don't know but we have our theories. One fascinating study looked at sets of identical twins and showed the higher your vitamin D level the longer your telomeres were suggesting it may be something to do with ageing. When comparing the highest level of vitamin D with the lowest values, the difference in telomere length suggest this was equivalent to 5 years of life expectancy.

Am J Nutrition, 2007, Richards et al.

Well that's settled then, isn't it? If all I need is vitamin D then I am going to the supermarket to get some.

I saw it there in the vitamin aisle last week when I was shopping. I just have to be careful not to take too much.

Well unfortunately nothing in medicine ever seems to be quite that simple. There were 2 very detailed reviews of this topic in 2014, each showing different results. Up to now there has been a general consensus that if you are vitamin D deficient then replacement therapy is associated with a lower risk of breaking bones and falling over, as it improves both muscle strength and bone strength. That seems to be where the consensus ends. The first review looked at 95 scientific studies involving about 900,000 people and this included randomised placebo controlled trials. They showed low levels of vitamin D were associated with many of the diseases mentioned and that supplementation seemed to reduce the risk of mortality amongst older adults by about 11% when vitamin D3 was used.

The other study was a similar review, including 107 systematic literature reviews and 161 meta-analyses (mind boggling numbers of patients!) and they concluded that "highly convincing evidence of a clear role of vitamin D (supplementation) does not exist for any outcome." They even question if it is of any use preventing in bony fractures and falls in the elderly. They thought it was useless. Both reviews were published in the same edition of the journal below.

British Medical Journal, 2014, Theodoratou et al and Chowdhury et al.

Amazing isn't it, when looking at the same thing medical scientists come up with completely different answers. Probably the reason we not infrequently give our patients completely wrong advice.

If you are vitamin D deficient then short bursts of non-burning sun exposure would seem to be sensible and supplementation with vitamin D3 is not unreasonably but stick to the guidelines and don't take huge amounts. More is not always better. Your vitamin D levels will not "overdose" with sun exposure as your body carefully regulates this. Tablets don't.

Remember vitamin D may not be the reason for the effects described with sun exposure, there are other possibilities I have not discussed including melatonin. You were probably designed for a small amount of regular sun exposure – but be careful not to get burnt. You get adequate vitamin D levels with about 10-15 minutes of sunlight three times per week but this time figure is dependent on latitude, altitude and the colour of your skin. More than about 15 minutes does not give you more vitamin D as it reaches a steady state in the skin, where the sun is breaking the vitamin D down as fast as it is producing it.

Sorry if I have left you a bit confused here, but we don't know all the answers. Should I still avoid the sun to minimise my risk of dying from melanoma or not? I hear you asking. The last thing I want here is children or adolescents ignoring current guidelines and getting sunburnt on my advice. Where older people are concerned however I think they should make an effort to get limited sun exposure – not sunburn.

Let us look at this another way. Using Australian statistics, which are by no means comparable with the European studies above, but do give you a different perspective. In Australia, 30% of all deaths in men and women are from cardiovascular disease. Just over 45,000 Australians died from this in 2015. In 2016 (I can't find the 2015 figures) there are estimated to have been 1774 deaths from melanoma and I am assuming roughly the same number of Australians between 2015 and 2016. This is 3.8% of all cancer deaths. This equates to one Australian dying every 6 hours from melanoma and one every 12 minutes from cardiovascular disease. The terrifying thing about melanoma is many of those who die are younger. In Australia melanoma is the number one cause of cancer related death in under 30-year old's, something I do not want you to forget.

What must to realise from these figures however is that melanoma deaths are relatively uncommon compared to cardiovascular deaths. No matter how tragic the circumstances of a death, when you are dead you are dead. If you take 1000 dying people, 300 odd will die from cardiovascular disease in Australia. Sun exposure potentially reduces this to 200, saving 100 lives according to the European data I have presented to you. This is conservative as the studies above suggest a reduction in all-cause mortality of 30% or 300 lives with sun exposure, not 100. At a guess if this sun exposure doubled or tripled the death rate from melanoma it may go up from 5 to 10-15 lives lost. The sun exposure has then saved 85-90 net lives, in this guestimate for want of a better word. Remember these are not official figures or official recommendations.

In summary, I don't want anyone getting sunburnt and I do not want children or adolescents to be more sun exposed and ignoring guidelines. When it comes to the rest of you however some sun exposure may not be as bad a thing as you have been led to believe. The sun is not evil, it may be your best friend.

CHAPTER 11

The Moon

I am using the moon here to signify sleep or at least sleep duration in a 24 hours' cycle. Life has evolved on the planet of ours with the planet spinning and taking 24 hours to complete a cycle. This gives us very roughly 12 hours of daylight and 12 hours of night. Almost all multicellular forms of life have adapted their life to this cycle with sleep or something resembling this. When you start messing around with this proven formula for life things begin to go wrong. Your lifespan and health span suffer as a result.

The Japanese were one of the first groups to recognise this. In the economic boom of the 1980s it was go, go, go and sleep was one thing you had to do without. Workers began dropping dead from "karoshi" which was their term for overwork. They were having sudden cardiovascular events including heart attacks and strokes.

American surveys for sleep duration reported at least

one third of people were getting less than 6 hours' sleep, the average being 6.8 hours which is apparently down by 1.5 hours on 100 years ago. About 20% of Americans are subjected to shift work with significant implications for their sleep.

So, what is all the fuss? I don't need much sleep! Well apparently, you do. Sleep is not overrated.

It doesn't matter if you are a fruit fly, a mouse, a rat, a dog or a human. If you start with a fruit fly and alter its genes so it thinks it doesn't need much sleep (like macho men above) you also dramatically shorten its life. If you keep a rat constantly awake it dies within 2-3 weeks, as do dogs and mice. In animal models, long term sleep deprivation results in negative effects on their hormones, their metabolic function, their immune function and their life expectancy.

Now as previously discussed you cannot do these types of studies in humans but you can look at healthy young "volunteers" like medical students and subject them to partial sleep deprivation. Especially if they want to pass their exams. If you do this they display impaired glucose tolerance or insulin resistance, higher levels of the stress hormone cortisol, increased activation of the sympathetic nervous system resulting in higher blood pressure and heart rate, reductions in the hormone leptin and increases in the hormone ghrelin both of which serve to increase appetite. There are also changes in immune function with increases in inflammatory messengers (IL-1B, TNF-alpha, IL-6 and all serum immunoglobulins) with the subsequent imbalance likely to promote inflammation in the body. There is also a reduction in the body's ability to clear damaging free radicals from the brain, the liver and the heart, resulting in potential damage to the cells and the DNA in these cells (animal studies – not medical students). So you can see where all this is leading...

Sleep: A Health Imperative, SLEEP, 2012, Luyster et al.

Sleep is not just something to fill in time waiting for the sun to rise. It is very important for proper functioning of an organism. In mammals and birds, we divide the sleep into 2 main phases, rapid eye movement (REM) and non-rapid eye movement (NREM) sleep. The NREM if further divided into 3 phases with the deepest sleep being the third of these termed N3. This deep sleep is said to be restorative and associated with marked reduction in output from the sympathetic nervous system with falls in blood pressure, heart rate and slow stable breathing. It takes about 60-90 minutes to get to this N3 part and typically you cycle through REM and NREM cycles 4-6 times per night, cycling once every 90-110 minutes. If you interfere with this N3 and shorten it there is an increased cardiovascular disease risk. If you actively try to resist sleep your brain begins imposing "micro-sleeps" on you which may last 3-30 seconds and which you are unaware of. Not good if you are driving a car at high speed. This certainly may shorten life and not just yours.

Deep within the centre of your brain, is the suprachiasmatic nucleus, where your internal clock is located dictating your circadian rhythm. It is influenced by light input from your eyes but even without this its internal pacemaker will produce a roughly 24-hour rhythm of sleep and wakefulness. This circadian timing system influences many other bodily functions including your body temperature, and hormones such as melatonin (which promotes sleep) and cortisol. When you mess with this system with jet lag or with shift work or chronic sleep deprivation this results in negative effects in metabolic function, cardiovascular disease, cancer progression and mortality risk.

The cardiovascular effects of sleep deprivation have been shown in multiple studies. 7-8 hours is the amount of sleep associated with the lowest risk for cardiovascular disease or death, both of which increase when one goes above or below this figure. In an American study of just under 7000 adults followed for 9 years, if they slept less than 6 hours or more than 9 they were at 70% increased risk of death during this period from all-causes. Another study showed if they got less than 4 hours sleep men were nearly 3 times more likely to die within 6 years of follow up compared to those sleeping 7-7.9 hours. Sleeping more than 10 hours roughly doubled mortality (1.8 times). Both these studies confirmed the U-shaped curve for mortality, predominantly from cardiovascular disease.

Sleep 1983, Wingard et al, Arch Gen Psychiatry 1979 Kripke et al.

The metabolic issues are also well documented in many studies showing a strong link between disordered sleep, obesity and type 2 diabetes. Sleeping less than 5 hours per night has been shown to increase the odds of obesity by a factor of 1.5 times per hour of sleep deprivation. Again, this is a U-shaped curve for obesity and diabetes with studies showing increased risk for both short and long sleep duration but more pronounced with short sleep. The Lowest predicted BMI is at 7.7 hours sleep.

Plos Med 2004, Taheri.

There is also data linking short sleep duration to cancer, particularly breast cancer, uterine cancer, colorectal cancer and prostate cancer. Women sleeping greater than 9 hours possibly have a reduced risks of breast cancer. The mechanism is not clearly understood but presumably may relate to insulin resistance and all that follows as these are some of the primary cancers increased with mTOR stimulation and the metabolic syndrome. I am assuming the study groups were matched for weight. These cancers are also more common in shift workers.

B J Cancer 2008 Kakizaki et al, Cancer 2010 Thompson et al.

Accidents and sudden death speak for themselves when working with excessive daytime fatigue and sleepiness when operating machinery or driving a motor vehicle and up to 20% of road traffic accidents are felt to relate to this issue. The implications for society as a whole are very significant.

Now when we are talking of sleep it is not just the duration we are interested in, it is also the quality. You cannot just lie in bed and look at the ceiling. Remember the sleep which is most important here is the deepest stage of NREM sleep or N3. The hardest to get to. That is when everything gets reset and the sympathetic (fight or flight) part of your nervous system gets turned down, lowering blood pressure and heart rate. If you don't sleep long enough you never get there and as a result will feel lousy and possibly more anxious the next day.

This is what happens with sleep apnoea or "sleep disordered breathing" which is becoming very common in our increasingly obese society. What happens is simple. As people fall asleep with this condition they obstruct their airway with the swollen tissues in their throat, including their tongue which is markedly enlarged and filled with fat. The result is the level of the oxygen in their blood stream plummets and the brain urgently wakes them up again to tell them to breathe. The alternative is to die. They go through this cycle of sleep wake multiple times every hour and they never achieve deep sleep. If you have 30 sleep apnoea cycles per hour, each lasting 2 minutes it is a bit hard to get to that elusive N3 deep sleep part of NREM (which may take more than 60min to achieve).

The result is not good. It is estimated that up to 20 % of the population suffer from this condition and less than 25% of those with severe disease are diagnosed and treated.

In a study in Wisconsin 1522 people were followed for 18 years. Sleep disordered breathing (SDB) or sleep apnoea of moderate severity was associated with an all-cause mortality increase of 300% or 3 times when compared with individuals with no SDB, if severe SDB this figure was 3.8 times. The risk of cardiovascular mortality was increased a whopping 5.2 times – that is greater than 500%. These results show that untreated SDB or sleep apnoea syndrome is associated with a high mortality. Other studies have shown strong associations for risk factors for cardiovascular death such as high blood pressure and features of the metabolic syndrome such as insulin resistance. It is postulated that this relates to reduced melatonin secretion with subsequent increased sympathetic nervous system activity but we don't have firm data to fully understand what actually causes the increased risk of death.

Sleep, 2008, Young et al.

So, it is settled then, the moon is important too, but you should not be lying awake looking at it.

CHAPTER 12

Psychological influences on ageing

As I subtly tell my patients, when I get the response; "are you saying this is all in my head?" the only effective way of separating the head from the body is with a guillotine. Mind and body are very closely interrelated and affect one another in countless ways. Sleep is an example already given. If you go messing around with the internal clock deep in your brain there are serious metabolic consequences for the rest of your body affecting your heart, liver, pancreas, immune system... and consequently possibly the length of your life.

It is not surprising then that how you feel about yourself is also important. Measuring emotions is a bit messier than a simple blood test to measure a hormone level and a bit harder to reproduce. It is done with questionnaires essentially just asking "how do you feel"

Subjective wellbeing is further broken down into three parts, these include your satisfaction with life (Evaluative wellbeing), your happiness or sadness in life (Hedonic wellbeing) and your sense of purpose and meaning in life (Eudemonic wellbeing).

Having a sense of purpose in life or so called eudemonic wellbeing was looked at in an English study.

They followed 9050 people with a mean age of 64.5 years for 8.5 years after completing their questionnaires. During this time 1542 of the group died. They divided the participants into four groups essentially measuring the purpose in life scored from 1-4. The death rates for the quartiles with increasing life purpose (from lowest to highest score for purpose in life) were 29.3%, 17.5%, 13.4% and 9.3% over this time. This is a dramatically different result, suggesting if you have little purpose in life you are three times more likely to die than someone who feels they have a purpose. Clearly there are numerous other factors which may have contributed to this thinking but if you do not have a purpose for life you had better go out and find one while you still can. Charity work and caring for others is a good start. Go after your dreams!

The lancet. Nov 2014, Steptoe et al.

What about your mood or your hedonic wellbeing? Does it matter if you feel depressed or unhappy? Well it probably does. A systematic review of 70 studies investigating mortality in healthy and physically diseased populations suggests that a positive psychological wellbeing or affect (mood) was associated with a reduction in mortality from cardiovascular disease in healthy and diseased groups, the effect being greatest in the healthy disease free group at about 18% reduced risk of death. There were a lot of studies looked at here but most of these were from 15 or more years ago and looking at cardiac patients predominantly. They all tended to show an association however with increased depressive scores correlating with increased risk of death. A better way of looking at this would be that a positive outlook and mood decreases your risk of death.

Psychosom Med, Sept 2008 Childa et al.

The same groups above have reviewed the effect of having a religion or spirituality with risk of death in review of 69 studies. Overall there was a positive effect with an 18% reduction in death if you were religious/ spiritual compared to those who were not but this was only shown in disease free people. In those with physical disease it seemed not to impact on survival. They also warn the results should be interpreted with caution because of the presence of publication biases, in other words those who had positive studies publishing them when those with negative studies did not, so you potentially only got one side of the argument.

Psychother Psychosom 2009 Childa et al.

The bottom line would appear to be, it is beneficial to have a purpose in life, to be positive about life and spirituality may help. Much of this is about doing things with other people, for other people, and having a close network of friends. Those friends are important, hang on to them.

CHAPTER 13

Long lived communities and what they have in common

This issue has been discussed and researched at length by Dan Buettner, the author of "The Blue Zones" books and if interested you should read these as they make some very pertinent observations. He and his researchers have been to the communities who seem to live the longest and observed their lifestyle and diet to try and sort out what it is that leads to their longer lifespan when compared to most of our modern societies, what do they have in common?

He has then taken the "lessons" back to communities in Europe and the USA and been able to demonstrate a drop-in disease rates and markers of cardiovascular disease such as serum cholesterol and blood pressure. It is a bit early to be able to show reduced mortality.

He summarises his work with nine lessons for longevity. These are:

1. Move naturally, don't overdo it with exercise such as pumping iron.

2. Have a purpose in life, a reason for getting out of bed

3. Relax, shed stress, chill out.

4. Eat less. Stop eating when you are 80% full, not when you cannot physically fit anything more in your stomach.

5. Eat less meat, get your protein from plant sources such as beans and lentils

6. Drink in moderation. Seventh day Adventists don't drink at all but most of the other long lived communities do drink 1-2 glasses of wine per day, usually red.

7. Have a faith. This is a common trait in these people. The denomination does not matter.

8. Love others, particularly family and partners and keep ageing parents and grandparents close.

9. Stay social, they all tend to have good social networks to support one another

I think he deserves a round of applause for this common-sense approach and following this advice is likely to be beneficial for all of us. I will review this when I summarise my views in the final chapter of this book with my additions and clarifications.

The communities discussed include;

- Mountain Villages in the island of Sardinia in Italy. This area holds the world record for men reaching the age of 100

- The Okinawa Islands of Japan

- Loma Linda, California where a group of Seventh-day Adventists are living and formed the study group.

- Nicoya Peninsula, Costa Rica

- Some communities in Sweden and you could possibly add the Kitava Island off New Guinea

- The Islands of Ikaria in Greece have the highest percentage of people living to over 90 year of age on the planet. 1/3 of their population make it to their 90s with almost no dementia.

They are clearly not identical in their lifestyles but they do share a number of things which Dan Buettner has attempted to summarise in the list of 9 rules.

Their lifestyles tend to be more relaxed and less rushed. Moderate physical activity is part of life. There is a purpose for getting out of bed in the morning. They eat less and what they do eat is largely plant based. They don't drink to excess and they engage in religion or spirituality, family life and social life.

Interestingly some do smoke but less than the rates in our society.

The issue he has not stressed here is they all tend to work outside in sunny environments and will have had large amounts of sun exposure. Sun screen is a relatively recent thing, so it was not available when they were young and I doubt they even use it once they get to old age. All the communities excepting Sweden are relatively close to the equator and many of the groups live at altitude, again increasing relative UV exposure.

Looking at their diets none are particularly low in carbohydrate averaging about 65% of calories from carbohydrate, often root vegetables like sweet potatoes and from legumes like beans and lentils. Not from processed forms of carbohydrate. They tend all to be thin and exercise regularly and if tested are very likely to be relatively insulin sensitive, in which case carbohydrate should not be harmful. Remember if insulin levels are low they will not stimulate mTOR.

Fats made up 20% of their calories, usually from mono-unsaturated sources like olive oil. Those on the island of Kitava do consume a moderate amount of saturated fat from coconuts without apparent harm.

They all consume relatively low amounts of protein and I think this is critically important, with 15% or less of their calories from protein and this is usually plant based. If they had animal protein it may only have been 1 or 2 times per week and in moderation. The exception was the Pescotarian Seventh-day Adventists who ate a small amount of fish daily, usually salmon. Remember amino acids from animal sources contain the highest levels of branched chain amino acids which stimulate mTOR the most effectively. It surprises me that the Pescotarian out lived the vegans in this group of Seventh-day Adventists but this was a small study and the data needs to be reproduced in other studies to be sure it is correct.

I think the protein intake is likely to be the most important issue here but staying thin with regular exercise and sunshine exposure is also likely to be important and emotional/social/psychological issues cannot be discounted but are harder to measure.

I doubt you will find a long-lived group of humans or insects anywhere on this planet who eat a diet very high in animal protein. It also clearly helps to exercise and stay thin.

So, what do the majority of us do in Western society? We eat a very high animal protein diet, we are obese or over weight and we don't exercise. Except to get off the couch to get another beer out of the fridge while watching the footy! We also stay out of the Sun preferring to watch TV indoors. No wonder we are all having open heart surgery in our 50s and dying in our 70s.

You couldn't get it more wrong if you tried.

CHAPTER 14

Bringing it all together for a long and healthy life

Now I apologise for all the figures and references in this book, the aim is not to confuse or overwhelm you, I just know that if I was the one reading the book I would not accept many of the statements I have made without the evidence to back them up. If you disagree with any of my conclusions you can look up the journal articles on which they are based and make conclusions of your own. This chapter is short and simple with recommendations to follow if you want to maximise your health span and avoid disease. The potential to avoid premature death, or if you like increasing your lifespan, is thrown in as well at no extra charge but remains a side issue.

The other issue which upsets some readers is my writing style. Some have called it "direct" or "unedited." Attacking the customer or reader, even if partly in jest is not a very good formula for success, and I stress my comments are only partly in jest. The books are not written for financial success. They don't make money. They are written for patient education and to make a difference. If you have stayed with the book to this section then there is hope for you. Those of you who threw the book out at the first perceived insult were unlikely to take any of it on board anyway, they were presumably more concerned with their own fragile egos.

I don't apologise for slapping you in the face or alternatively on the backside. Unfortunately, it is more often the latter as I find most of you have your heads stuck in the sand. If you get a fright or a shock at what you are reading you are much more likely to remember the content and hopefully act on this, rather than just fall asleep and not even remember where you were up to in the book. Your remembering the content of the book is my aim and why I write in a relatively direct fashion.

So how do you stay healthy, avoid disease and doctors. Well there are no guarantees for any of us. The unexpected may well be just around the corner. I am just suggesting you give yourself the best chance of living a long healthy life. That you put the right oil in your engine.

My suggestions are:

1. Do not eat a lot of animal based protein. I think this is much more harmful to your health than you

have been led to believe. If possible get your protein from plant sources such as beans and lentils but you will have to do a bit more reading if you are going to make this purely from plant sources to be certain you get all the essential amino acids. I would be aiming for no more than 0.5g per kg of lean body mass if using animal protein. I would do this by including small amounts of seafood or dairy in your predominantly plant based diet. Remember the animal protein is the garnish on the side of a meal, not the main event. This will be controversial but is likely to be one of the most important issues.

2. Eat lots of Vegetables. This is to be the mainstay of your diet. Not just any vegetables but the more colourful the better. Mix the colours. mTOR does not like those colours particularly the reds, blues and purples as they tend to shut it down. Variety is good, the more different vegetables the better but I would avoid bland high carb vegetable such as regular potatoes. Eat orange or purple sweet potatoes instead if you eat root vegetables and look for those purple carrots.

3. If you are, or are likely to become, insulin resistant, a direction most of the population is currently heading, then carbohydrates and to a lesser extent protein are not good for you. You are living in a state of carbohydrate poisoning. You should avoid starchy vegetables such as potatoes, all grains and all added or concentrated sugars including fruit juice. Never

replace carbohydrate with protein, use healthy fats or oils and eat lots of vegetables. Your body can turn protein into carbohydrate and both will stimulate the release of insulin, the very thing you are trying to avoid if you want to live longer, remain healthy and lose weight. You can have small amounts of fruits but some are better than others such as berries and watermelon. If you are thin and insulin sensitive you can eat carbohydrate freely. Consider reading the book "Death by Carbs" to give you more advice about where to find carbohydrate and how to avoid it if you are obese or overweight.

4. Avoid large amounts of saturated fats including animal and plant based saturated fats such as palm oil or coconut oil. Eat as much polyunsaturated and monounsaturated fat as you like. Again remember processed foods are loaded with palm oil and should be avoided. Saturated fats seem to push you down the road to the metabolic syndrome, particularly when eaten with carbohydrate. This syndrome potentially ends in premature death.

5. If the food is processed forget it. You should not eat processed foods, they contain large amounts of sugar, dangerous saturated vegetable fats and emulsifiers which worsen your insulin resistance or diabetes. Make meals yourself or get others to do this for you. Do not use anything that comes in containers of any sort unless you have carefully read the ingredients. This includes processed sauces, tins, and virtually anything

in a packet. Even things like that soft spreadable butter or ice cream are likely to contain emulsifiers which are potentially very bad for you and your gut, your liver, your cardiovascular system and consequently your quality and quantity of life.

6. Once you are an adult regular controlled sun exposure should be considered. You do increase your risk of skin cancers potentially including the dreaded melanoma but your overall risk of death from other causes is probably many times higher if you stay indoors. Sunburn is not to be recommended, you cannot catch up in large exposures. You must do this regularly in smaller amounts – measured in minutes not hours. Wear sunglasses to avoid cataracts. This will be controversial but I feel the data is there to support this approach and it is important.

7. Get enough high-quality sleep, you are aiming for 7-8 hours per night. If you cannot sleep see your doctor or try various relaxation exercises or more physical exercise in the mornings. If you are likely to have diseases interfering with sleep like sleep apnoea then see a doctor and get treatment. Dropping dead may be the alternative so get help while you still can.

8. Make regular physical exercise part of your life. Within reason the more the better in terms of preventing disease, particularly short bursts of intense exercise. Huge amounts of exercise such as running marathons daily is likely to do more harm than good in terms of

heart damage so be sensible. Weight bearing/lifting exercise is important as you age, so only swimming in a pool or walking around a golf course is not ideal. Neither is yoga in isolation.

9. Medication and supplements. Once you get to middle age, and possibly before, you should discuss taking Metformin with your doctor. As I have stated the evidence of benefit in non-diabetic people is not there yet but the protective effect in cancer, cardiovascular disease and dementia is clearly not related to diabetic control – it is a different effect, likely applicable to all including non-diabetics. The dose is whatever you can take without side effects being an issue for you, likely somewhere between 500 and 1500 mg daily. The slow release formulation may be better tolerated. Don't take over 2 g daily and if you have kidney problems make sure you address this with your doctor first. This drug has been around for a very long time and would appear to be very safe. There may be studies in the future to show you have wasted your time taking it but it is unlikely to do you any harm. If you don't take it and it is subsequently proven to be beneficial to non-diabetics you may have missed out on the potential benefit. If it does prevent or delay dementia developing for example this may be a very significant benefit. It is very unlikely we can reverse dementia once it has set in.

Aspirin should be considered as well at 100mg daily. If you are taking a proton pump inhibitor for reflux up to 600mg per day should be safe but there is always a small risk of inducing a gastric ulcer. There is some evidence the anticancer effect of aspirin is dose dependent, in other words the more the better. Taking aspirin is not without risk however and you need to understand the risks

If you take other supplements make them mTOR inhibitors so at least there is a theoretical reason for taking them. You can get tablets and capsules of resveratrol and curcumin for example both of which we know inhibit mTOR but make them from trustworthy sources. Alternatively use spices such as turmeric, chilli and others generously in your cooking. Make the food as colourful as possible. Eat the NMN.

Nicotinamide mononucleotide (NMN) and or Nicotinamide Riboside (NR) as described in chapter 6 hold very real potential for benefit. I would be watching this space carefully as it will hit the mainstream media soon. If proven beneficial in humans I would give them serious consideration. I would have a low threshold for taking them now but I cannot recommend the general public using them widely at this time because of the potential risks, not as yet clarified and we do not know the optimal dose. Those mice took huge doses. Remember the story of Vitamin A and lung cancer in smokers? That seemed like a good idea at the time too.

10.   Be happy. Easier said than done I know but happiness is often related to other people so get out and mingle with them. Join clubs, help others, and make a point of smiling at others in this world. You are likely to get much more in return.

11.   Have a purpose in life. If you haven't got one start setting yourself goals. One of the most rewarding things for people to do is to help others by joining a charity. Find a reason to get out of bed in the morning. Even looking after a pet is a good start.

12.   Drink alcohol in moderation. 1-2 glasses per day, preferably of wine translates to a lower risk of dying than not drinking.

13.   Drink coffee regularly, full strength coffee none of this decaffeinated rubbish. If you don't like coffee keep at it until you do! Green tea is an alternative but it contains much less caffeine when prepared. Caffeine is a potent mTOR inhibitor and should be part of your life if you can tolerate it.

Now there are some things here which will attract a lot of criticism from my learned medical colleagues and other groups such as dieticians and public health advocates. They are those who are more conservative than I in making recommendations and would like these things proven in proper blinded randomised medical trials before giving an opinion to the public.

I am on their side in this respect — I would love to know the results of these high-quality studies, it would make giving advice much easier and I would be able to sleep more peacefully. The problem is we do not have these studies to guide us and it may well be many years before we do. The answer once we do have it firmly embedded in rock may no longer be relevant to you anymore.

It is not likely any of the recommendations above will cause harm. We are currently experiencing a crisis in public health issues, particularly obesity, the metabolic syndrome and all that goes with it. Someone has to do something. We have the absolutely ludicrous situation where drug companies are rushing for example trying to market more very expensive drugs to treat things like fatty liver disease! Why not? Governments will pay for the tablets and these drug companies stand to make many more billions of dollars, predominantly from your taxes. No one seems to want to say the truth which is simple. If you stop eating too much carbohydrate, and to a lesser extent protein, you will cure fatty liver disease in the majority of patients! Even without exercise. No drugs required. No cost to taxpayers or health departments. Simple dietary change. No need to go hungry.

Surely, we can spend some time and energy educating people how not to get sick in the first place, rather than picking up all the pieces at great personal and financial cost when they do?

What ever happened to simple common sense?

The most controversial recommendation here is related to sun exposure. I stress I would strongly advise against ever getting sunburnt as this is more strongly associated with melanoma. Similarly, I make no recommendations for increased sun exposure for children and adolescents. Non-melanoma skin cancer however is less likely to be life threatening and more easily treatable than a heart attack or a stroke.

The studies we have to date suggest that the health benefit with some sun exposure, coming mainly from reduction in cardiovascular disease risk, may exceed the potential harm from all forms of skin cancer by more than 10/1. You do the maths, you read the articles and you decide what is right for you. I for one will not be avoiding intermittent non-burning sun exposure. Vitamin D tablets just don't seem to cut it, so it must be something else about the sun conveying this potential benefit. Remember the Mediterranean factor may not be anything to do with diet at all.

The next issue which will generate criticism relates to suggested dietary changes. No one wants to change guidelines once they are in place. The more they are repeated the more "correct" they become. Right? No, I don't think so. Again, you read the literature. When you are young, growing and having or feeding children protein is fine. Once you get past this time it likely shortens your life and I would cut down your protein intake. The possible exception is old age where muscle strength is very important to independence, but then again so is the absence of dementia so I am not sure what the answer is here. More protein may worsen dementia. In general terms, most of us eat far more protein than we need, at least in my opinion.

The third issue, likely to generate scathing criticism is suggesting you take the medication Metformin not of proven benefit in non- diabetic individuals. The evidence is on the table suggesting it may be beneficial. The question then becomes is it likely to do any harm? I think the answer to this is no. This drug has been used for 60-70 odd years, surely if there was something very bad about it we would have worked it out by now, wouldn't we?

I'm sure there are better drugs coming, which will prevent ageing and disease and may well replace things like Metformin. As medical science advances, we will gain better understanding of the issues related to ageing and disease and there will be new advice given. At this time, these things are "future prospects" only.

The advice above is based on what we know now. What you can do now. If you follow this advice I think you will be potentially much better off, you will avoid some of the disease burden from which we suffer in our society, and you will need to see much less of the medical profession as a result.

You are likely to have a longer health span and life span.

Only you can do it. As they say; "Talk is cheap" so get off your backside, stop talking and start acting.